T0380926

COMFORTING YOUR UNCOMFORTABLE STOMACH

A Companion for Silent Sufferers of Nausea and Vomiting

LAURA A. DOTSON
KENNETH L. KOCH, M.D.

Archway Publishing books may be ordered through booksellers or by contacting:

Archway Publishing
1663 Liberty Drive
Bloomington, IN 47403
www.archwaypublishing.com
844-669-3957

ISBN: 978-1-6657-1874-5 (sc)
ISBN: 978-1-6657-1876-9 (hc)
ISBN: 978-1-6657-1875-2 (e)

Library of Congress Control Number: 2022902679

Print information available on the last page.

Archway Publishing rev. date: 08/30/2022

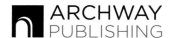

Comforting Your Uncomfortable Stomach is a must-read for those suffering from nausea and vomiting. This book answers many of the questions that patients often have regarding the whys and hows of the way the digestive system works and why the patient may experience nausea and vomiting. It continues to provide an easy-to-follow, three-step diet with wonderful and adaptable recipes in order to help mitigate the symptoms. The content is easily understood, and the artful graphics complement the physiology and recipes included. The authors understand what patients experience, and the result is an outstanding and highly beneficial book filled with hope. I highly recommend *Comforting Your Uncomfortable Stomach* to anyone who may be suffering from nausea and vomiting. If you want to learn, understand, and become empowered to help yourself, this book is for you.

Maryangela DeGrazia-DiTucci
President | Patient | Founder
Association of Gastrointestinal Motility Disorders, Inc.
www.agmdhope.org

This book is dedicated to all of you who suffer in silence! You are the brave, indomitable souls who will survive these maladies! The work to support yourself is worth it! I know you. I am you. I promise to work tirelessly to support you! Silence no more!

Laura A. Dotson

This book is dedicated to my wife, Elizabeth, for decades of support and to my patients with chronic nausea and vomiting. My patients taught me not only how they chose foods to decrease their nausea and vomiting but also how they suffer, how they want their lives back, and how they cope and carry on.

Kenneth L. Koch, MD

Contents

Foreword

The terms *comforting* and *companion* are not generally associated with nausea and vomiting. However, they are perfect in describing Laura Dotson and Dr. Kenneth Koch, not only as individuals but also as writers. In *Comforting Your Uncomfortable, Stomach*, they provide a practical guide for those struggling with debilitating disturbances of digestion. I understand that disturbance personally as a fellow sufferer from gastroparesis. This companion guide is a lifeline for those who suffer and for those who love them as well. I only wish it had been available at the start of my journey!

Prior to suffering from chronic nausea and vomiting, food was at the center of my social life. From girls' night out to romantic evenings and vacations, the plans always centered upon an excellent food choice. Birthday parties, baby showers, and special events left the ultimate decision of whether to cater the menu or do potluck. Then, along comes a disease that no one in my world had ever even heard of that caused incessant vomiting, constant nausea, and rapid loss of one hundred pounds and changed my social life drastically. How do you attend events when the smell of food makes the nausea worse? How do you explain to family and friends that the eating regimen you figured out doesn't include the *special dish* they made for you without being offensive? How do you accept invitations to special events when you know that a cost is associated with your RSVP, and you are uncertain of how you will feel on that day? Social interactions were only a small portion of my life changes with the onset of sickness.

The weakness that ensues due to an inability to digest is an unfathomable experience to some but an all-too-common experience to many. It is still heartbreaking to recall the pain in the eyes of loved ones as they stared at me with such pity and fear while I continued to lose weight. I was given tons of home remedies to stop the vomiting and rid the nausea—from the well-known crackers and ginger ale to the unheard-of trick of licking salt from the palm of my hand. I didn't find relief until I tried Dr. Koch's *Three Step Diet* solution outlined in this companion guide. Grappling with the physical aspects and finding understanding is key. Knowledge gives so much power.

My journey was a little different from most. Gaining that power—that knowledge—took a very long time. I didn't have any of the risk factors that would lead to the diagnosis of gastroparesis or in the direction of a gastric-emptying study. All I knew was that I was sick. I couldn't stop throwing up. I was constantly nauseous. It literally felt like we were fighting a battle in the dark. I was losing weight for some unknown reason. When I was finally diagnosed, understanding it and managing it proved to be equally difficult. Getting properly diagnosed felt like I just put a name on a disease at first. My husband and I did a great deal of research online. He made all kinds of smoothies, removed things from my diet, and did his best to create an eating plan for me. Eventually, I was referred to Dr. Kenneth Koch.

My initial visit with Dr. Koch lasted a couple hours. It was probably the most comprehensive first appointment I had ever had with a doctor. He patiently answered every question I had and even repeated his answers for my mom when she asked the same questions. He provided so much comfort. I left feeling empowered because I had answers. I understood the digestive system. I understood what was happening within my body. I had a plan. I had the *Three Step Diet* to try. Though that was only a first step in what would be a long journey, it was light in a dark situation. It brought peace of mind, and it brought hope.

Like me, Laura Dotson suffered with chronic nausea. She understands the importance of hope, the importance of peace, the importance of knowledge, and the importance of a plan when you are battling digestive disturbances. Together with Dr. Koch, she is packaging the necessities to bring light to the fight into this companion guide to equip the reader with the tools to manage digestive disturbances. The guide is providing the reader with understanding of the digestive system, diseases and disorders, coping skills, and diet. Instead of searching multiple websites and listening to multiple podcasts, all the information can be found in one central location. How awesome is that?!

Suffering with something as intrusive as chronic nausea can be debilitating not only physically but emotionally. The writers left no stone unturned as they also addressed psychological components.

Reading this, I imagine all the people I can share this with in explaining why my stomach hurts and how they can help. I imagine the people who have followed my blog I can recommend this to. I imagine my children's friends and their parents who want to understand more about their mom. I imagine friends at church, neighbors, and others who want to learn more. I imagine the person who is suffering in silence and doesn't want to talk about it to whom I can lend a helping hand in the form of *Comforting Your Uncomfortable Stomach*. This book is a game changer and a lifeline. Comforting companion!

Ronetta D. Graham, MAED, LCMHC, NCC

What is a companion book for silent sufferers of nausea and vomiting? And why in the world would anyone choose such an odd topic about which to write a book? Taboo discussion! Gross! Yuck! And all other expletives!

The reason is simple, yet the silence on this subject is deafening within the general public. There is an astounding and pervasive presence of nausea and vomiting permeating all groups of people. A recent review of the burden of gastrointestinal diseases in the United States from 2016 showed that nausea and vomiting were the number two and three leading gastrointestinal diagnoses that prompted the patient's visit to the doctor. There were 3.9 million visits for nausea and 5.4 million visits for vomiting. The number one symptom for office visits was abdominal pain, and there were 19 million visits. The causes of nausea and vomiting are numerous and often unknown and long-lasting. Most people with nausea and vomiting, especially long-term nausea, suffer alone. A social life is unimaginable to them because of their symptoms and embarrassment. Sufferers' self-image can erode, and hopelessness can ensue.

The countless number of you experiencing the debilitating symptoms of nausea and vomiting were likely flooded with relief when you saw this book. Finally, someone has broached the subject about which none of us is comfortable talking. Likely, you had no idea so many others suffer like you. As children, we were taught bodily functions like nausea and vomiting are inappropriate to speak of outside the home. Our mothers taught us that. The authors are here to debunk that notion. It is imperative to have conversations with others about your nausea and vomiting. Don't hide it! It is vital for you to educate others about your experience and your resulting emotions. Your suffering is beyond what most people can imagine enduring. Speaking out will help them realize they know someone who suffers like you. You are not alone. You absolutely do not have to suffer silently.

Comforting Your Uncomfortable Stomach is a unique collaboration born from an authentic relationship between a world-renowned gastroenterologist and his once very sick patient. Kenneth L. Koch, MD, and Laura A. Dotson have collaborated to provide you guidance and direction from both the physician and patient perspectives. You will read Dr. Koch's approach to choosing what to eat when you are nauseated. His entire career has been dedicated to understanding, reducing, and even eliminating nausea and vomiting. You will also find recipes Laura A. Dotson developed when she was in his care and extremely ill from gastroparesis. The book provides details for you to consider in talking with your doctor about your symptoms and concerns. You will have access to a glossary of medical terms to help you describe your symptoms to your doctor. These definitions will also help you understand the diagnoses and tests your doctor discusses with you. This companion is here to diminish your suffering in all aspects of your life.

Preface

Introduction to Patient and Physician

Laura A. Dotson

Several times in my life, I have read the research of John Fabre, a French naturalist from the early twentieth century. He conducted an experiment with pine processionary caterpillars, which blindly follow the caterpillar in front in a head-to-toe formation. Fabre carefully arranged the caterpillars in a complete circle around the rim of a flowerpot in which he had placed pine needles—their main sustenance.

The caterpillars followed each other around the rim of the flowerpot for seven days. Eventually, each of them dropped dead of starvation. They had each been so focused on following the one in front that they did not recognize the life-sustaining nourishment just inches away. These caterpillars made the ultimate sacrifice because they did not choose to explore options. They did not consider a new way to deal with their predicament.

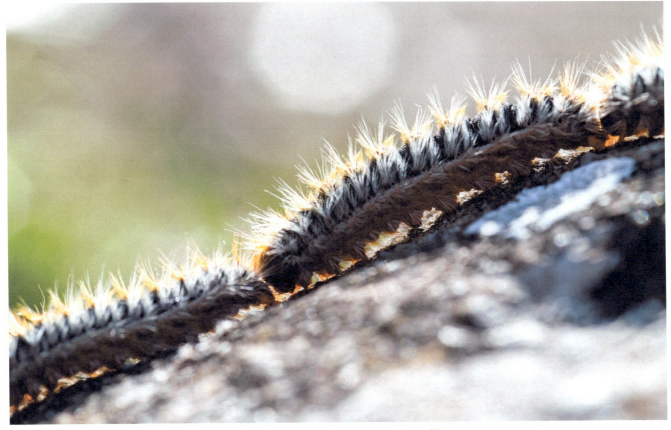

Fabre's processionary caterpillars

Far into my journey to stop my severe nausea and vomiting, I ran across Fabre's work again. This research had an entirely new meaning to me. At that time, I was following the instructions of a doctor who was not helping me. Fabre renewed my determination to flourish and regain responsibility for my own healing. I was literally so sick of being sick that I was desperate to investigate anything that could provide nourishment to all of me. I dove into the flowerpot to save my livelihood and literally my life. I became a student of my symptoms. I read everything I could get my hands on to educate myself on the possibilities of *why* and *what* to do.

My nausea and vomiting began immediately after I had my gallbladder removed. My mother had told me, "Eating will be different from now on." The conversation ended there. We did not delve into what she really meant by that at the time. This was a sad and stressful time in my family given the recent, premature death of my beloved sister, Robin, at age 49. As I recall, I did not want to even think about food. I had been hyperconscious for 17 years that she could not eat or drink. Two brain aneurysms had left her unable to swallow and totally dependent on tube feedings. No birthday cakes. No traditional Thanksgiving foods. No favorite Christmas goodies. My heart hurt for her continually.

I also assumed my nausea and frequent vomiting were what my mother spoke of as being different, and my digestive system needed to readjust after my gallbladder operation. Ironically, when she was in her early pregnancy with me, my mother thought her nausea was related to her gallbladder. Also ironically, my mother's death was caused by the inability to eat from aspiration pneumonia. I cannot express the absolute power with which these two women persevered through suffering based on faith and love. The gorgeous connection I had with both is ever present in my mind and joyfully leads my path daily.

I went to the post-op visit with my general surgeon and told him I was still vomiting. His comment verbatim was, "What do you mean *still*?" He promptly sent me to a local gastroenterologist. This gastroenterologist prescribed drugs for acid reflux. I was persistently telling him I did not believe my issue was acid reflux, and the medications were not providing relief, comfort, or hope. I was not heard. I was coldly ignored. This went on for many months.

He seemingly had no respect for my body wisdom or empathy for my debilitating symptoms. He did not know what my symptoms could tell, and the worst insult was that he had no desire to listen to me. However, I had options instead of following him around the rim of the flowerpot. Trust your body wisdom—your gut. Find anyone and everyone who will listen to you. It is crucial for your healing and may become so in someone else's healing.

Even at eight months after the gallbladder operation, I was throwing up everything I ingested. It was obvious no further digestion had occurred past my mouth. Most days I vomited thirty-five to forty times. I was scared, confused, and angry, and I was having a difficult time carrying on any degree of a normal life. No one was listening to me. It was as if I was living in some parallel universe, and no one could see how I was suffering.

I lost weight, and people complimented me. I did not want that. I wanted *me* back. I began to hide my weight loss because people at work knew I was vomiting. With no diagnosis, coworkers and friends naturally concluded I was not being truthful and had an eating disorder. It became necessary for me to always carry plastic bags and tissue. I drastically decreased my time away from home. Everything that makes me Laura was dwindling away. I had no idea what to do.

The inattention sparked my spunk, and I dove into the pine needles again. I went to see another local gastroenterologist of whom I had heard great things. She also happened to be my client at the time. She listened to *me* in our first discussion. Based on the symptoms I described, she ordered the appropriate test immediately.

The test she ordered is called a gastric emptying test. I easily ate some Eggbeaters™ along with toast and jam that had a small amount of radiation in them. I remember thinking they tasted so good and tried to stay focused on not being nauseated. I knew this test needed to be completed.

After the four-hour observation, those tasty, precious eggs, toast, and jam had not moved through my stomach at all. Over that time period, they should have been out of my stomach and in my intestines with their nutrients absorbed into my body for energy.

This drastic halt of progression of food emptying from the stomach is called gastroparesis. *What?* I had never even heard the word or known one other person with it. My high school Latin helped me to understand it meant my stomach was paralyzed. The second gastroenterologist knew an expert on this disease at Wake Forest Baptist Medical Center, named Kenneth L. Koch, MD. Filled with hope once again, I immediately scheduled a visit with him.

At my first appointment, Dr. Koch reviewed my symptoms and test results. He confirmed my diagnosis of gastroparesis and explained all the treatment options available. He gently told me there was no cure, and he would be with me to make me as comfortable as possible. Dr. Koch began by emphasizing that food choices can help decrease nausea that occurs after eating. He went over in detail his *Three Step Diet for Nausea and Vomiting*, which he told me he learned from talking with thousands of patients. He talked about how the stomach is a sophisticated muscle that mills food, but my stomach was very weak or paralyzed. Milling was disturbed. The *Three Step Diet* took my stomach's weakness into account and the foods within each step are easier for my weak stomach to receive, mill, and empty. By choosing these foods, nausea caused by the stomach can be decreased.

Even as I began following his plan, my physical and mental stamina were rapidly waning. I felt a sensation of my muscles literally pulling away from my bones. Even though I had been a physically strong person, I would get winded walking from the house to the car. The first antinausea medication I took made me extremely drowsy. My wonderful mother came to live with me to drive me around for work. I had my Gatorade™ and chicken broth in the back seat while also still carrying the plastic bags for unpredictable, frequent vomiting. My mother was plagued with guilt for eating in front of me. At that point, my insurance did not cover Zofran for gastroparesis. Prior to my employer becoming self-insured, my out-of-pocket cost every month was in excess of $3,000 almost twenty years ago. That is another book, huh?

Every time I felt myself becoming dehydrated, I would use all my energy to drive to Wake Forest Baptist Medical Center Emergency Department where Dr. Koch had established a protocol for rehydrating his patients. I had no idea it would be so easy. When the triage nurse asked how he or she could help, I would say, "My name is Laura Dotson. I have gastroparesis, and I am a patient of Dr. Koch's. I have vomited thirty-six times today."

Every single time, the response was, "OK, Ms. Dotson, let's get you back and get you hydrated so you can go home." They were listening, too!

I was receiving encouragement and wonderful care from valet parking to Dr. Koch. I ate foods within his diet yet longed for more taste and flavor. I could feel my life passing before me. I knew I had to do something more. I was not about to die on the rim of the flowerpot.

So, I got to work. I read everything I could about nutrition, vitamins, minerals, etc. I began adding other nutrients to my chicken broth and pureeing them, sometimes more than once. I would strain purees through cheese cloth. Every time I went back to Dr. Koch for a visit, I would take some samples of my new recipes for his taste and digestive approval. Together, we realized many patients with nausea and vomiting could benefit from these recipes. The recipes have few ingredients and are designed for multiple servings for later use. By preference, I use only organic, locally grown foods and filtered water. This practice eliminates unnecessary, unknown chemicals, hormones, or ingredients. I have no idea the effect they may have on my body, so I choose not to ingest them.

I am beyond grateful to have found Dr. Koch. He was open to any ideas I brought to the table to regain strength in all areas of my life. When I proposed options with which I wanted to experiment, such as massage and acupuncture, he would say, "Use your intuition to do what you need to heal." Can you imagine? A highly educated, world-renowned gastroenterologist standing inside the hallowed halls of a traditional medical institute using the word *intuition*. I knew I had been divinely led to the physician who would support me in getting my life back. And indeed, he did. I have been eating a regular diet for more than a decade. I endearingly refer to him as the *guru of gastroparesis*. I am grateful he remains my advocate and gastroenterologist to this day.

My sincere desire by sharing what we both have learned in my healing process is that you will have a guide that I did not. I know you will be able to build a strong, healthy life despite the current bump in the road you are experiencing. There is so much hope in the rapidly progressing field of medicine. Do all the research you can, and do not hesitate to tell others what you are experiencing. That person may also be a silent sufferer.

Kenneth L. Koch, M.D.

Comforting Your Uncomfortable Stomach is a resource for those who suffer with nausea and vomiting. They are remarkably common symptoms. For instance, 98 percent of the population has experienced nausea. Forty-three percent reported nausea symptoms on more than one occasion in the past three months. More than 50 percent of the population choose to self-treat their nausea with over-the-counter products, and 12 percent do so by eating crackers and drinking ginger ale. For most people, nausea strikes and then just goes away. However, in 2018 there were 2.2 million emergency department visits for nausea and vomiting, which is twice as many as for gastrointestinal bleeding. Many of you have chronic nausea and vomiting. Most likely you have seen your doctor, been referred to specialists, and undergone many tests. Drug treatments for nausea are often minimally helpful, especially if the cause remains unexplained.

In many cases even with a specific treatment for nausea you may still have some nausea every day. It is at these times that you may not know what to eat or if you should eat at all. Very few patients with chronic nausea have had dietary instruction for how to eat when they are nauseated. Ingesting most foods when you are nauseated may make you even more nauseated. This especially occurs if your stomach is not working properly as we discuss in the book. Nausea and vomiting often lead to dehydration that may require visits to the emergency department for intravenous fluids.

This book is designed to help you prepare for visits with your doctor, understand your gastrointestinal tract, learn the many causes of nausea and vomiting, and know how your stomach works. When you understand how the normal stomach works, then the three-step nausea and vomiting diet will make sense and you can use it to hydrate and nourish yourself. When nausea and vomiting is the issue, patients have many questions:

- How do I discuss these symptoms with my doctor?
- What is the cause of my nausea?
- Is there a treatment for my nausea?
- How does my stomach work?
- What do you mean my stomach is a muscle?
- What should I try to eat?

Nausea is a symptom that can be caused by many diseases and disorders. Therefore, it is important to try to obtain a diagnosis that explains the specific cause that is driving the nausea. Standard tests often come back with a normal result. Special tests of electrical and muscular function of the stomach may be needed to make a diagnosis. If a cause can be identified, then hopefully a specific treatment can be provided to reduce symptoms. My hope is that if nausea is eliminated, then vomiting disappears altogether.

A strategy to reduce nausea and vomiting is choosing the right foods to eat. To do this I have found that it helps if patients both understand how the stomach receives, mixes, and empties food and then choose what foods to eat using the *Three Step Diet*. The steps start with liquids that are easy to empty and progress to solids selected because they are easy for the stomach to mill and empty. The special recipes in this book that were created by Laura when she was suffering from chronic nausea follow the physiological principles of stomach emptying. I have listened to my patients talk about the foods they eat that did not evoke nausea or evoked less nausea. These food choices made sense to me based on gastric emptying, and I summarized them in the *Three Step Diet*, a diet that helped patients hydrate and maintain or gain weight.

I hope this book will broaden the choices of foods you will tolerate and enjoy, even if you suffer from nausea. The three-step diet encourages you to assess how your stomach *feels* during the day and select foods from step 1, 2, or 3 that seem right to you at that time.

Patients have told me over the years: "I just want my life back." It took me a long time to understand what this meant. An underappreciated aspect of chronic nausea and vomiting is that you tend to suffer alone. Others may be completely unaware you are suffering— possibly because you are hiding it—but your family and friends are the very ones who wish they could help you. They feel bad because you cannot enjoy the same foods they may be eating. You may have withdrawn from friends and family, especially at mealtimes because you fear your nausea will worsen. More deeply than I appreciated, our lives are *centered* upon sharing meals in solidarity—in togetherness with family and friends. Algernon Cash wrote in *Winston-Salem Monthly* magazine, "Food is love. It requires sacrifice, it unites, and it brings comfort." To be able to enjoy eating again with family and friends is the life my patients want back.

As you work to return to health, I hope the information in this book and the diet approach helps you select nourishment wisely to comfort your uncomfortable stomach.

In the first chapter, Laura and I discuss aspects of the doctor-and-patient relationship. Especially important is a relationship that is built on mutual trust and respect. Such a relationship helps the efforts of the patient and doctor to find specific diagnoses and helpful treatments.

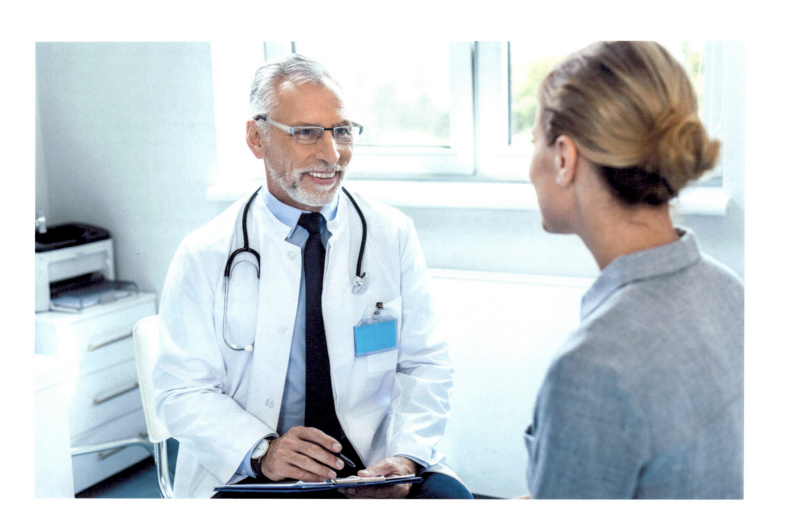

CHAPTER 1

Doctor and Patient Relate

The good physician treats the disease; the great physician treats the patient who has the disease.   William Osler, MD.

Dr. Osler was one of the founders of Johns Hopkins Hospital and is often called the father of internal medicine.

At the heart of good medicine is the harmonious relationship between doctor and patient—a relationship of mutual respect and care. Effective communication is the foundation of building this relationship. Trust and clear communication—listening and responding—are the keystones of high-quality health care. The breakdown in doctor-patient communication is the source of much patient dissatisfaction. This breakdown can begin because some patients have difficulty describing their symptoms and unmet needs. It can also occur because some doctors overestimate their ability to communicate the status of the workup, test results, next steps, or the fact that they care.

The relationship between doctor and patient has evolved over thousands of years. In ancient Egypt (4000–1000 BC), doctors used magic spells and natural remedies like honey and copper salts. Illness was thought to come from the wrath of the gods. The roles of doctor and priest were often filled by the same person who would use his unique skills to heal patients with offerings, concoctions, aromas, and tattoos to calm or drive away the god who sent the illness.

Hippocrates was a famous physician and teacher who lived in ancient Greece. He is considered the father of medicine. His Hippocratic Oath established an ethical code for doctors. Hippocrates died in 375 BC, but the oath is taken today by every new doctor graduating from medical school. During the time of Hippocrates, the Greeks developed a system of medicine based on evidence from observation and treatments using trial-and-error approaches. They no longer relied on magic and religious answers to relieve suffering. Hippocrates also wrote about diet regimens that would benefit his patients and is quoted as saying, "Let food be thy medicine and medicine be thy food." This book is dedicated to helping patients with nausea select foods that will nourish them while also decreasing their symptoms.

The Hippocratic Oath also represented a shift in the doctor-patient relationship. The oath obligated the doctor's responsibility to do no harm and to respect the patient's person and privacy.

Good doctor-patient relationships begin and continue with good communication. Good communication requires truthful talking and careful listening by both parties. Dr. Osler had this advice for doctors: "Listen to your patient; he is telling you the diagnosis." Careful listening to the patient's symptoms results in better diagnoses by the physician and better outcomes for the patient. Osler believed in the physician-patient conversation. This is how a successful office visit should be experienced. As discussed below, the patient and doctor bring different perspectives to an office visit.

Patient Perspective, Laura A. Dotson

How many of us go to the doctor with an internal plea to just *fix me*? We are living in a time when we get immediate satisfaction in all areas of our lives: Amazon next-day delivery, home grocery delivery, telemedicine appointments, and remote starters in vehicles. We must remember that a visit with the doctor is not like a trip to the auto mechanic. He or she does not simply plug in your big toe, and a list of diagnoses comes up on a screen. While there are many technologically advanced tests that can be performed, your doctor needs to hear the experiences that brought you to the office. Your diagnosis and comfort will be based on his or her ability to understand what you are feeling. Approach your doctor as an equal partner in your health care while maintaining ultimate responsibility for your own health. Do not forget: it is *your* life, and you can do anything.

Dr. Koch and I share a doctor-patient relationship based on mutual respect. I am dependent upon him to listen to my symptoms and experiences. He is dependent upon me to be as precise as I can be in communicating how I feel. This allows him to engage his knowledge and experience toward easing my *dis*-ease. The mutual respect present during my illness continues as we work to share our experiences with you in this book.

Doctor Perspective, Kenneth L. Koch, MD

I am a gastroenterologist who has studied nausea and vomiting and tried to help patients with these symptoms for many years. In addition to the suffering inherent in the experience of nausea and vomiting, the wonderful social interactions during mealtime are reduced or completely lost. It is understandable for a degree of depression to accompany these symptoms as the quality of life you have known diminishes. The journey of evaluation and treatment may be long. If that is the case, then the doctor and the patient can become frustrated. Good communication is the foundation for finding the cause for your symptoms and a helpful treatment.

After introducing myself, I usually ask about hometown, occupation, and family when I am meeting a patient for the first time. I then ask the patient to describe the symptom that bothers him or her the most. We then go over that symptom in detail: when it began, timing, relation to eating, factors that relieve the symptom, and so on. We review medications, operations, family and social history, and other medical issues. Tests that have been completed elsewhere are reviewed. A physical examination is performed. A list of possible diagnoses is prepared, and tests to prove or exclude the diagnoses are discussed. If the results of standard tests are normal, I order tests of the neuromuscular function of the stomach, esophagus, gallbladder, and small intestine as indicated. These tests are described in chapter 4.

The second visit is when the results of the tests are discussed in relationship with the symptoms. Hopefully, a diagnosis or several diagnoses are identified, and diet and drug treatments can begin.

Many of my patients have symptoms like Laura's, and I start with dietary advice to reduce symptoms and improve hydration and nourishment. I explain the *Three Step Diet for Nausea and Vomiting* that is detailed in chapter 5. Laura's recipes helped her through her years with severe nausea and vomiting and provide flavorful, healthy, and satisfying nutrition that follow the *Three Step Diet* approach. I hope the recipes will help you too.

In this book, you will read about the many organs within your gastrointestinal system, how they work, and especially how the healthy stomach works after food is chewed and swallowed. The focus on normal and abnormal muscular functions of the stomach will help you understand why some foods evoke symptoms and others reduce your nausea and vomiting. By choosing foods that are *easy* on your stomach, your hydration and nutrition can be maintained or improved.

Preparing to See Your Doctor

The ultimate objective of any doctor-patient relationship is to comfort you by decreasing your symptoms and improving your health. Thus, it is important for you to prepare for the office visit so it is productive. A few tips are offered below:

- Your visit is scheduled for a limited time, so focus on one or two major concerns for the visit.
- What questions or concerns do you have? It helps to write them down.
- Be honest and thorough in communicating your symptoms and concerns.
- Work with your doctor. Be sure you understand any plans and agree with them.

One idea for the visit is to describe your two most bothersome symptoms. This will help you and your doctor focus on your main issues and concerns. You may want to keep a journal of your symptoms, highlighting the one(s) that bother you the most. As you do this, those that bother you the most will become evident. Keeping a journal may also relieve some stress as you observe and record how you feel.

Other items to prepare and bring to your visit might include the following:

- A list of medications you are currently taking
- A list of previous medications and self-treatments that failed to help your symptoms
- A copy of test results relevant to your symptoms

Also, you may ask a relative or close friend to accompany you to help you remember your conversation with your doctor. You will want to make sure you understand your current diagnosis, what tests need to be done, any new treatments, and the next steps. Once you get home, questions always seem to come up about what was said or agreed upon during the conversation with the doctor.

Dialog

To provide a sense of what a helpful conversation for both you and your doctor may be like, we have re-created a brief dialog like the one we shared during the first visit.

Dr. Koch: What symptoms do you want to discuss today?

Laura: It is a long story! I will try to make it brief. I had my gallbladder removed over a year ago, and since then I have been vomiting everything I eat. It is obvious nothing has happened to my food after I chewed it. I have been prescribed multiple acid-reducing medications with no relief. I feel like the doctor I was seeing did not listen to me. I finally went to another local gastroenterologist who suspected gastroparesis. I had a gastric emptying, test and based on the results, she sent me to you because of your expertise in treating this disease. What is it exactly?

Dr. Koch: Gastroparesis means that your stomach muscles are weak, so it mixes and empties what you eat too slowly and much slower compared with healthy people. Nausea and vomiting are symptoms associated with gastroparesis, but other stomach neuromuscular abnormalities and diseases can cause these symptoms too.

Laura: How did that happen? I have never even heard of anyone having this!

Dr. Koch: Gastroparesis is more common than most doctors appreciate. Unlike cancer or heart disease, you don't see any ads about it. It is also not well known by patients. It is associated with diabetes, but many of those patients have not heard of gastroparesis. I know you are not diabetic, but in most patients, we do not know the cause of gastroparesis. However, gastroparesis can also occur in patients with heartburn and chronic indigestion.

Laura: That is amazing! So, why do I have it, and what can we do? It has already changed my life so drastically. I want it gone! I am independent to a fault, but you tell me what to do, and I will do it. Because of the nausea, I do not go out very much. All I can do is work because I must. My mother is even driving me around because Phenergan makes me so sleepy. I literally come home from work and get straight into my bed in order to have energy for the next day. I am traditionally a physically strong person, but my stamina is waning fast. Will I just have to live with this?

Dr. Koch: We may not ever know why you developed gastroparesis, but I am going to work with you now to try to reduce and manage your symptoms. I hope you can return to your normal life as soon as possible. I will also review our *Three Step Diet* for you to try. This diet will show you how to choose foods that are easier for your weak stomach to mix and empty. You choose what you eat from step 1, 2, or 3 based on how nauseated you are during the day. There are several drugs that increase stomach contractions and may also help your symptoms.

Laura: No one ever described a diet for me. I will do anything to feel like me again! Before I take a drug, I want to know how it works, how I might feel, and what the side effects might be. I have taken so many that have not worked. How long will it take me to recover?

Dr. Koch: OK. We will go over the diet so you will understand the three steps and how they are related to your stomach muscular function. We will also review each drug before we try it. Recovery is variable and depends on the cause of the gastroparesis. For example, gastroparesis caused by drugs and viruses frequently improves over time, but this may take one or two years in some cases.

Laura: I have been stressed out completely from not being heard. I am exhausted from this life-altering situation. I am working to find anything to help. I have been trying to relieve my stress and fear with massage and acupuncture. How do you feel about that?

Dr. Koch: Stress certainly doesn't help gastroparesis. Acupuncture can help some patients with nausea and vomiting. I am not sure about the effect of massage on nausea, but it certainly would not hurt you and it may help. Chronic nausea and vomiting can lead to depression. Antianxiety drugs and low-dose antidepressants may help. We have several different approaches to try as we consider diagnostic tests, diet, and drugs to help you with these symptoms.

In summary, the doctor-patient relationship is the key in the successful management of your overall health. The doctor must never give up working to understand the cause of your nausea and vomiting and seeking treatments to relieve your suffering.

In the next chapter, we describe the location and function of the organs in the gastrointestinal system. These organs change the food we eat into nutrients that are absorbed in our bodies. The pleasant sensations we normally feel after eating begin the digestive processes that sustain life. Life is good when the gastrointestinal tract works smoothly—some might say even gorgeously.

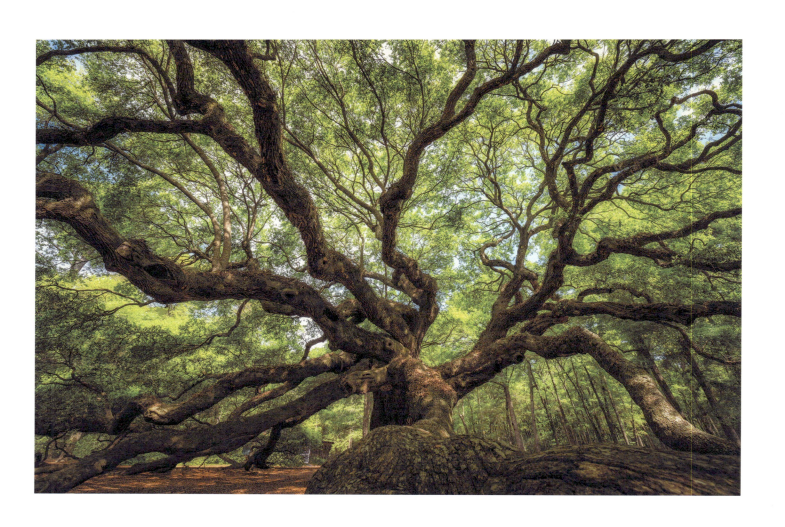

CHAPTER 2

Your Gorgeous Gastrointestinal System

Do you ever think about how your digestive system works? Most likely, you dream about what food might taste good but not about your amazing digestive system, which uses the food you eat to give you life. Digestion is a gorgeously sophisticated series of events that begins the moment you see, smell, or think about what you like to eat. These events do not stop until your body absorbs all the precious nutrients it needs and then rids itself of what you do not need.

Your digestive tract is a series of connected hollow muscular tubes and solid organs known as the gastrointestinal system (figure 2.1). Food moves from your mouth through your esophagus, to your stomach, along your very long small intestine, and through your colon. This amazing system efficiently processes everything you swallow to sustain your good health. It secretes enzymes and hormones, mixes and moves food, absorbs nutrients, and allows all that remains to exit your body. During most of this perfect process, you are not consciously in control—miraculous and amazing indeed.

Some of you may not like to think about anatomy per se or bodily functions. However, if you are suffering from nausea and vomiting and looking for answers, it is necessary to know what may be going on in your gastrointestinal system. Our description of the anatomy of your gastrointestinal system is meant to support you in your conversations with your doctor and your endeavors to get well.

Knowing as much as you can about your body is your best support in your journey with nausea and vomiting. In this chapter we will review how each organ of your digestive system normally works to process the food you eat into nutrients that can be absorbed and used by the body. Appreciating normal function will help you understand how you might develop nausea and vomiting. We will provide you with information so that you can be your own best advocate when you feel bad. You are not alone. Never stop searching for new answers and solutions. They come every day.

Mouth

The beginning of digestion can occur with the simple thought of food you enjoy. That thought travels across nerves from your brain to your salivary glands. They immediately begin to make saliva to prepare for the arrival of food and drink. When you put food in your mouth, your teeth tear and grind the food into smaller pieces. The salivary glands under your tongue and on the sides and roof of your mouth release as much as a quart of saliva each day. Saliva helps with swallowing, protects your teeth against bacteria, and aids in the digestion of food.

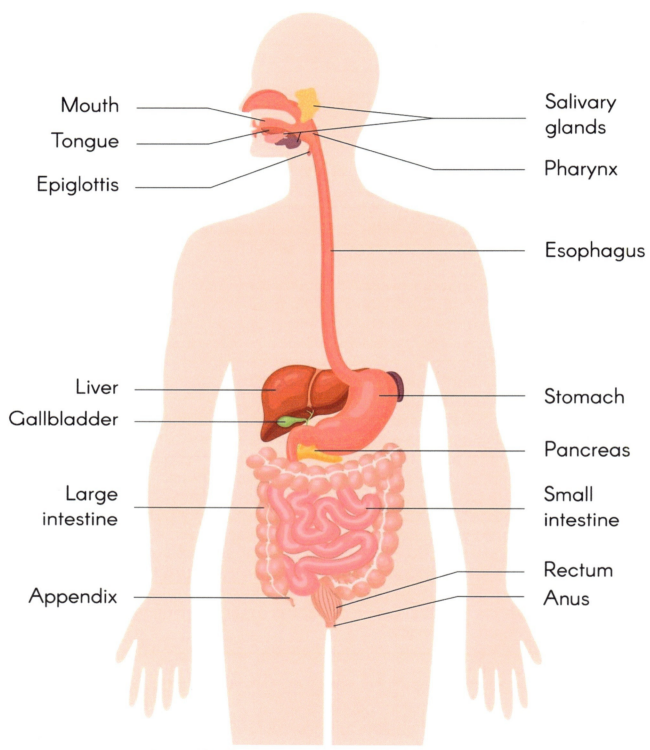

Mouth

Tongue

Epiglottis

Salivary glands

Pharynx

Esophagus

Liver

Gallbladder

Stomach

Pancreas

Large intestine

Small intestine

Appendix

Rectum

Anus

Figure 2.1: The gorgeous gastrointestinal system

Your teeth contribute to the beginning of digestion in a large way. As you chew, the different shapes of your teeth shred and grind your food. The very strong muscles in your tongue work with the teeth to form a soft, rounded amount of food for you to swallow. Up until the point you swallow, you are making conscious decisions about your food. However, once you swallow, the autonomic nervous system takes control. Your food first encounters a muscle called the upper esophageal sphincter. This sphincter opens to let the food from the mouth enter the esophagus. Sphincter muscles act like valves. They relax to let the precise amount of food and liquid pass down the tract. A sphincter muscle that you can watch is your pupil, the dark spot in the center of your eye. As the pupil responds to differing amounts of light, the muscle opens and closes to control the precise amount of light to reach the back of the eye. The sphincter muscles in your gastrointestinal system open and close in response to varying solids and liquids in a similar sensitive way.

Esophagus

When you swallow, the epiglottis covers the trachea to protect it, and the upper esophageal sphincter relaxes to allow food to pass safely into your upper esophagus. The esophagus is a tube of muscle about ten inches long and connects your throat to your stomach. Food does not just fall through the esophagus into the stomach. Each time you swallow, food is moved down the esophagus and into the stomach by contraction waves, which are the kind of contractions that are out of your control. Your digestive system has taken over.

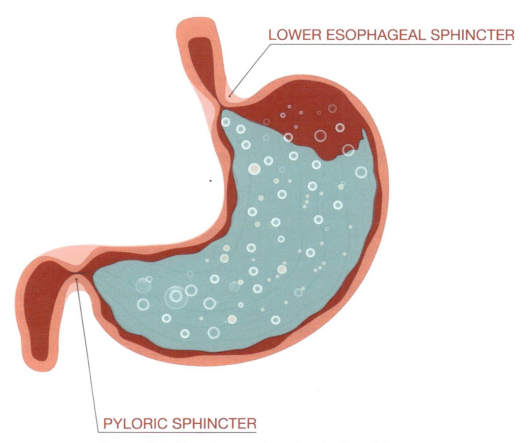

Figure 2.2: Esophageal and pyloric sphincters

9

Each time you swallow, the walls of the esophagus begin to move food to the stomach by gentle waves of muscular contraction. The esophageal muscle above the food contracts while the muscles below relax and allow the food to progress to your stomach. This process is called peristalsis and occurs throughout the gastrointestinal system. Just like at the top of the esophagus, there is also a sphincter muscle at the junction of your esophagus and stomach called the lower esophageal sphincter (figure 2.2). When your mouth and throat are not engaged in swallowing, this valve is closed to keep the acid in your stomach from coming up into the esophagus and causing heartburn. It is also the muscle that allows you to be unintentionally rude when air escapes with a burp.

Stomach

"My stomach hurts!" Well, exactly where and what is your stomach? Most of us refer to any part of our abdomen as our stomach. The stomach is just a small part of where a stomachache could be. Let's look at your anatomy to see what you might mean when you choose those words to describe what you are feeling.

Your stomach is a major digestive organ that secretes acid and does muscular work to break down food you eat. It is in the upper half of your abdomen, mostly on your left and central areas below the ribs (figure 2.1). It is a hotbed of complex nerve and muscle activity and is much more sophisticated than you imagine. Its initial muscle function is to relax in order to comfortably receive food you eat. We might take a clue and try to relax our entire bodies while we are eating instead of hurrying through a meal. Many cultures use their lunch as a time to relax and rest in order to work smarter afterward. Relaxation of your mind and body truly does aid in your digestion.

Second, the stomach gently mixes and mills those solid foods into tiny bits called chyme. The milling of food is helped by secretion of acid and pepsin by the stomach during the thought of food, the chewing of food, and the presence of food in the stomach. Mixing and milling are accomplished by coordinated waves of contractions that occur rhythmically every twenty seconds. These are the peristaltic waves, or contractions, of the stomach. This is indeed important muscular work since the proper milling of your food prepares it for emptying into your small intestine where even tinier nutrient bits are absorbed into your body to provide you energy.

While you are eating and shortly thereafter, you normally experience comfortable sensations as the stomach performs its work. In healthy people, hunger is often felt as emptiness in what's often called the pit of the stomach. Drinking liquid or eating solid foods reduces this hunger and replaces it with a sensation of comfortable fullness in the stomach. This comfortable feeling may last from minutes to hours depending on how much and what types of food you ate—protein, carbohydrate, or fat. We often call some foods *comfort food* because these soothing sensations can be felt not only in your stomach but over your whole body and mind.

The stomach requires an amazing amount of relaxation because your stomach is normally a small and collapsed muscular organ. The stomach gradually relaxes as it fills and increases in physical size to accommodate liquid or solid food you have eaten. Usually, we think of an increase in size being muscular work, not relaxation. This muscle relaxation occurs mainly in the upper part of the stomach called the fundus (figure 2.3). After receiving the food, the fundus gently pushes the food into the body and antrum areas of your stomach. The body and antrum work together like a gentle grain mill.

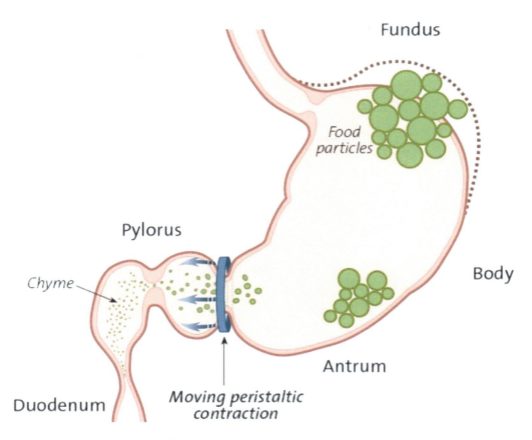

Figure 2.3: The stomach at work

When liquid nutrients, like those in a smoothie, enter the body and antrum areas of the stomach, very little milling and mixing is required. Solid food requires much more work to prepare it for the rest of the journey through your digestive tract. Each meal you eat offers different challenges and muscular work for your stomach.

With the help of gastric acid and digestive enzymes, the solid foods you eat are milled into chyme. The milling by the gastric peristaltic contractions occurs over many minutes, even hours, until all the tiny food particles are emptied from your stomach. During this phase of digestion, a single peristaltic wave will push less than a teaspoon of chyme out of your stomach through another sphincter called the pyloric sphincter and into your duodenum (figure 2.4). The pyloric sphincter helps to regulate the flow and volume of chyme the stomach empties with each peristaltic wave with the precision of a Swiss watch.

The stomach's peristaltic contractions are so critical that they are paced, much like the way your heart contractions are paced. Have you ever considered the heart and the stomach to be such close cousins? Your stomach has a natural, built-in pacemaker system just like your heart (figure 2.4). We usually think of a pacemaker as a mechanical device implanted to stimulate normal rhythms of the heartbeat. Your stomach's pacemaker rhythm comes from special cells located in the pacemaker region. The electrical pacemaker signal moves along the body and toward the antrum at an average rate of three cycles per minute (cpm)—much slower than the heart. Your stomach's pacemaker cells control the frequency and speed of gastric peristaltic waves that mill and empty chyme into your duodenum.

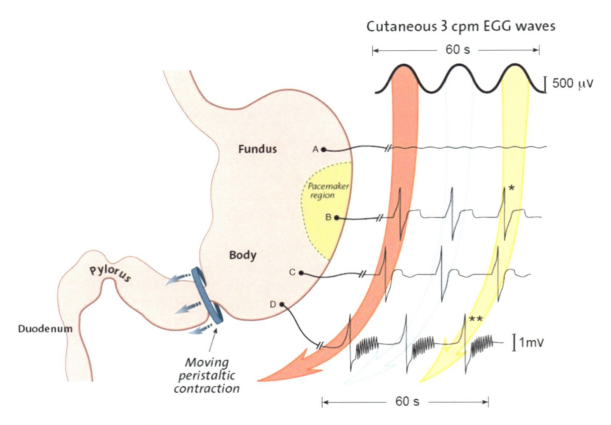

Figure 2.4: Peristaltic stomach contractions and electrical rhythms

The pacemaker region is shown shaded in green. The letters A, B, C, and D represent electrodes surgically sewn onto the stomach to record electrical events from the pacemaker and muscle cells. These electrical events are also recorded through electrodes placed on the skin of the abdomen over the stomach. This recording is called an EGG, or electrogastrogram.

Other factors that affect the electrical rhythm of your stomach include:
- vagus nerve activity
- insulin and blood glucose levels
- sympathetic nervous system activity
- gastrointestinal hormones

Like they say, "You are what you eat," and the work of the stomach is required for this nutritional truism.

Small Intestine

Chyme, the finely mixed and milled food you ingested, is gently and rhythmically emptied into the small intestine through the pyloric sphincter. It is further broken down and then absorbed throughout the twenty feet of this muscular tube. These tiny nutrients are absorbed and transported to the liver to be made into fuel and building blocks of the body. The small intestine has three parts: the duodenum, the jejunum, and the ileum (figure 2.5).

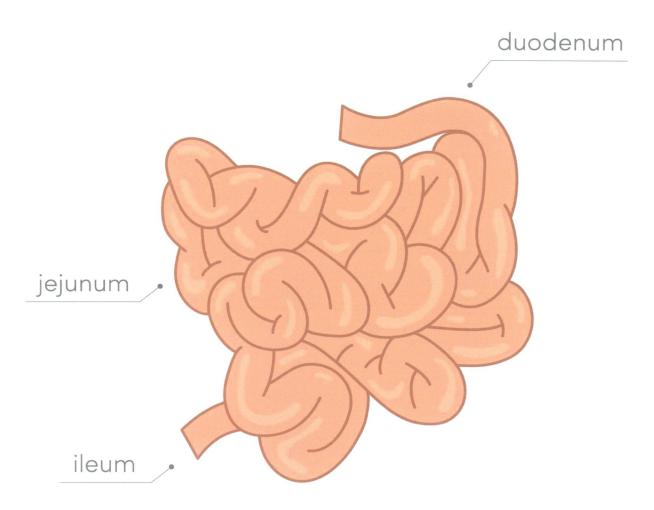

duodenum

jejunum

ileum

Figure 2.5: The small intestine

The duodenum is part of the small intestine closest to the stomach where the intense breakdown of food continues. It is an amazing junction where chemicals from your pancreas, liver, and gallbladder meet with the purpose of further breaking down the chyme. The results of this breakdown are nutrients (e.g., glucose, amino acids, fatty acids) that are absorbed by the remaining areas of your small intestine.

The jejunum is a high-action spot. This is the place where those perfect nutrients are absorbed. Peristalsis is slow here, and nutrients may travel only several inches so they can be absorbed. The word *jejunum* is derived from the Latin word *jejunus*, which means "empty of food." It is usually found empty within hours after a meal because it efficiently absorbs the nutrients.

The ileum is the final section of the small intestine and is about three feet long. It specializes in absorbing bile acids and returning them to the liver for recycling. The lining of the muscular wall of the ileum and the jejunum consists of a series of folds, each of which has tiny, fingerlike projections known as villi. These villi absorb the nutrients. At the end of the ileum is another sphincter called the ileocecal valve. This sphincter controls the flow of fluids and undigestible fibers into the cecum of the colon. The valve also prevents the backflow of colon contents into the ileum.

Pancreas

Your pancreas is a soft gland located just behind your stomach. It's about the size of your hand. Some say it looks like the shape of a fish. The pancreas is a unique organ because it has both an endocrine and an exocrine function. Endocrine glands secrete hormones directly into the bloodstream. The islet cells of the pancreas secrete hormones that serve as chemical messengers to help regulate blood sugar levels, appetite, and stomach emptying. The exocrine glands of the pancreas secrete enzymes for digestion directly into the duodenum. Pancreatic enzymes travel through your pancreas via ducts and flow into the upper part of your small intestine called the duodenum. Each day, your pancreas makes and secretes about 30 ounces of digestive juice filled with these enzymes. They allow the nutrients you ingest to be completely absorbed by breaking down sugars, fats, and starches.

There are several pancreatic hormones and enzymes you should know about, including:

- *Insulin* is the hormone released into the blood when your blood sugar, or glucose, level goes up. Insulin helps glucose enter the body's cells where it can be used for energy or stored for future use. If the pancreas is not able to deliver enough insulin, over time your blood sugar levels rise, and you develop diabetes.
- *Glucagon* is the hormone that regulates your use of sugar already in your body. If your blood sugar gets too low, glucagon helps raise it by sending a message to release stored sugar from your liver and your muscle tissue.
- *Amylin* is a hormone that helps control appetite and stomach emptying. Additionally, it helps manage your blood sugar after you eat by suppressing your pancreas's production of glucagon. This intricate balancing act enables you to maintain normal glucose levels and energy throughout the day and night.
- *Lipase* works together with bile from your liver to break down fat in your diet. If you don't have enough lipase, your body will have trouble absorbing fat and the important fat-soluble vitamins. Symptoms of poor fat absorption include diarrhea and fatty bowel movements.
- *Proteases* break down proteins in your diet. These enzymes also help protect you from germs that may live in your intestines, like certain bacteria and yeast. Undigested proteins can cause allergic reactions in some people.
- *Amylase* helps break down starches into sugar (glucose) your body uses for energy. If you do not have enough amylase, you may get diarrhea from undigested carbohydrates.

Liver

The liver is the largest internal organ in the human body. Weighing about three pounds, the liver is reddish-brown in color and feels rubbery to the touch. The liver has two sections, called the right and the left lobes. The smaller of the two lobes lies above the stomach, and the right lobe lies beneath the ribs. The right lobe is located under your right rib cage for its protection. They are separated by the falciform ligament, which attaches the liver to the front of the body wall. This vital organ performs hundreds of functions, and requires nutrients to do so. Nutrients are the digestive products of the healthy foods you eat. Here are just a few of those liver functions:

- Albumin: The liver produces this protein, which carries hormones, enzymes, and vitamins through your bloodstream.
- Bile: The liver produces bile, which aids in the digestion and absorption of fats in the small intestine.
- Blood: The liver filters all the blood from the gastrointestinal tract, gallbladder, and pancreas and removes toxins and harmful substances.
- Blood clotting: The liver aids in blood clotting by producing coagulation factors like thrombin and other proteins involved in the breakdown of clots.
- Glucose: The liver processes glucose in two ways. It removes excess glucose (sugar) from the bloodstream and stores it as glycogen. As needed, it can convert glycogen back into glucose.
- Immunity: As part of the filtering process, the liver removes bad bacteria from the GI tract.
- Vitamins: The liver makes bile, which is needed to absorb vitamins A, D, E, and K, and stores these vitamins plus B12.

Gallbladder

The gallbladder is a small, translucent pouch that sits immediately under your liver. It is connected to the liver by bile ducts. The gallbladder stores bile that is produced by the liver until it is needed in your small intestine. After meals, the gallbladder is nearly empty, like a deflated balloon. Before a meal, the gallbladder may be full of bile and about the size of a small pear. When food enters the duodenum, the hormone cholecystokinin is released. Cholecystokinin signals the gallbladder to contract and empty stored bile into the common duct, a tiny muscular tube that enters the duodenum. Bile helps digest fats, but the gallbladder, as you know, has been deemed nonessential if it is inflamed as in cholecystitis. Typically, removal of your gallbladder causes minimal to no digestion issues. In some cases, diarrhea and fat malabsorption occur after the gallbladder is removed.

Appendix

The appendix is a finger-shaped organ, about three and a half inches long, and attached to the cecum which is in the lower right of your abdomen near your hip bone. The function of the appendix is unknown. It is thought to be an obsolete organ that played a more important role in that past than it does in modern times. Many of you have had appendicitis and had your appendix surgically removed.

Colon

The colon, or large intestine, is responsible for storing and eliminating all food your body is unable to absorb in the small intestine. While the colon, at three to four feet long, is much shorter than the small intestine, it is larger in diameter. The anatomical regions of the colon, as seen in figure 2.6, are the cecum, ascending, transverse, descending, sigmoid colon, and rectum. These regions appear to form just short of a complete box in which the length of your small intestine is nestled. Your ileocecal valve lies between your ileum and the cecum. At this point in digestion, what remains in the colon is water, plant fiber, and electrolytes. Peristaltic waves help the ascending colon absorb water and deliver contents to the transverse and descending colon.

While these undigested contents are in your colon, good bacteria continue to break them down. These billions of bacteria are called the microbiome. It is a topic of much discussion and research at present. Good nutrition helps to maintain your own good microbiome. The colon moves the non-absorbed materials and microbiome into the sigmoid colon, which serves as a storage-holder until the urge to have a bowel movement is sensed. Muscles in the rectum in coordination with the anal sphincters move stool out of the body through the anus. The journey of the food you eat, through your amazing digestive system, results in nourishment for your body. The journey is complete with a regular bowel movement.

This amazing conveyor belt of digestive tubes and organs—the gastrointestinal system—is intricately coordinated so that meetings among food, acids, enzymes, and hormones result in nutrients that can be absorbed. Electrical impulses along many nerves and pacemaker cells cause muscle contractions and relaxations of which we are not aware. We go on our way, comfortable after our meals, as these beautifully designed events sustain our lives.

In the next chapter, we review diseases and disorders that are associated with nausea and vomiting. From diseases outside the gastrointestinal system to obvious stomach ulcers to subtle electrical dysrhythmias, one or more of these problems could be driving your nausea and vomiting symptoms.

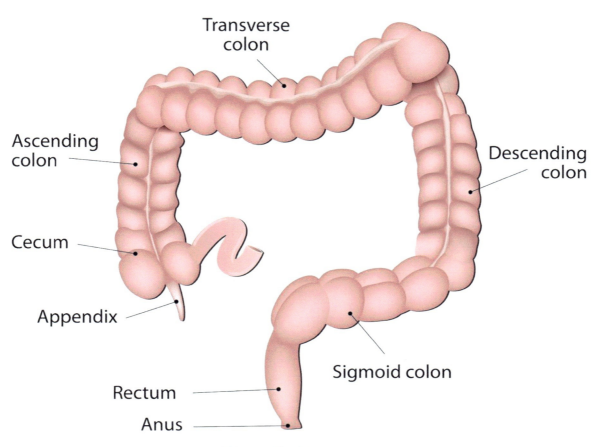

Transverse colon

Ascending colon

Descending colon

Cecum

Appendix

Sigmoid colon

Rectum

Anus

Figure 2.6 The colon

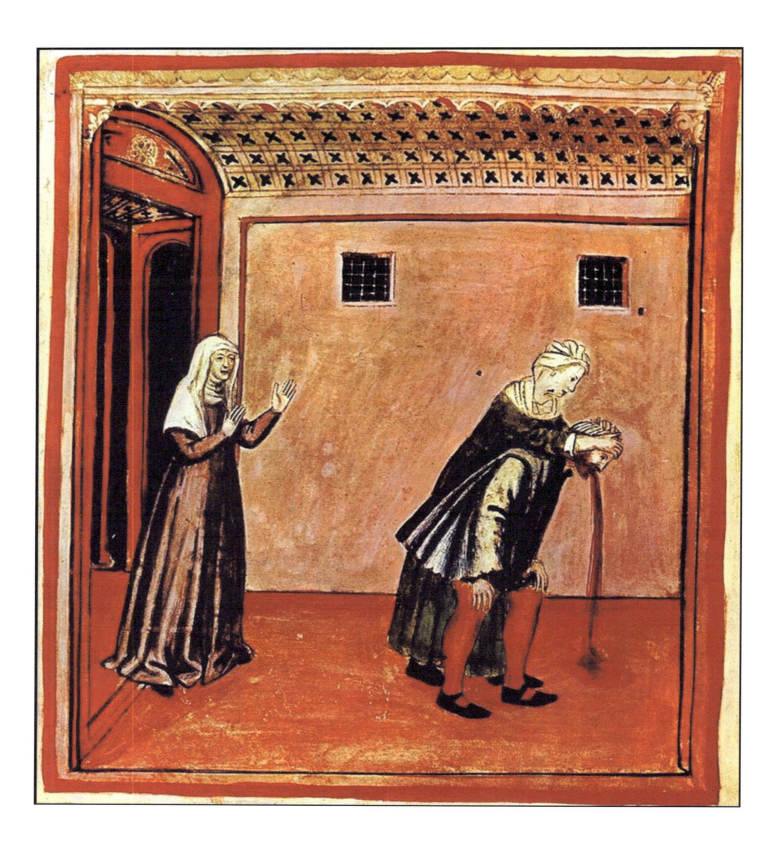

CHAPTER

3

The Be-*causes*

As you know all too well, nausea is an uncomfortable, queasy feeling that causes you to stop in your tracks. Nausea and vomiting can strike anywhere, anytime. When either or both strikes, you quickly begin to retrace your steps. You mentally list what you ate and with whom you've come into contact. Hopefully, you will only feel unlike yourself for a short while.

Each of us has felt squeamish from nervousness, excitement, or motion. Your stomach starts rumbling, and you begin swallowing a little harder. You might also feel some light-headedness, fatigue, and stomach discomfort or pain. The feeling of nausea is hard to describe because all of us feel it differently, and the nausea can arise from different organs. Regardless, vomiting may come next.

Nausea usually precedes vomiting, yet vomiting may occur without nausea, such as after extreme physical exertion. Vomiting is a reflex controlled by areas in the brain that prompt a series of strong contractions of the stomach. Severe dehydration and decreased urination can result if vomiting does not stop. If we have little or no nausea, then hopefully there will be no vomiting. In order to find relief, we usually search for remedies to eliminate nausea.

If all of us experience nausea and vomiting, why don't we know how to avoid it and stop it? The many sources of nausea make the cause hard to immediately determine. When you feel so yucky, you want to know why. What is the *cause* I cannot *be* myself?

Common Causes of Acute Nausea and Vomiting

Acute nausea and vomiting come on quickly, last several hours to two or three days, and then disappear. At the onset of symptoms, you do not know if it is going to be acute or long-lasting. All the causes of acute nausea and vomiting can become chronic, or long-lasting, so you want to monitor and track symptoms.

Nausea and vomiting are symptoms your body gives you to tell you something is not normal. You want to be aware of what brings it on and what gives you relief. Are there any other accompanying symptoms? Is there a pain? The cause of any pain should be determined. Keep notes in a calendar so you will be aware of recurrences. It is best to seek advice from a doctor if nausea, vomiting, and any other symptoms you are experiencing reoccur. Short-lasting nausea and vomiting can be caused by many conditions, and several are described below.

Viruses

The most common gastrointestinal viruses are the Norwalk virus and the Rotavirus. Both are highly contagious. These viruses cause gastroenteritis, which is inflammation of the lining of the stomach and intestinal tract. Nausea, vomiting, and diarrhea along with a low-grade fever and abdominal cramping can be severe. Many people with acute coronavirus infection (COVID-19) have nausea, vomiting, diarrhea, and respiratory symptoms. Gastroenteritis is sometimes referred to as the stomach flu. That can be confusing, as there is no influenza present. At the same time, if you do test positive for influenza, you may feel nauseated and vomit. Influenza and gastroenteritis are very different illnesses.

Nausea, vomiting, and diarrhea may lead to dehydration, especially in children and the elderly. It is vital to sip on electrolyte drinks to prevent severe cases of dehydration that may require hospitalization to receive intravenous (IV) fluids. However, for most people, gastroenteritis is a self-treated disease that lasts two to three days and then gradually disappears. Because these viruses are so highly contagious, you will want to isolate yourself or the patient from others for a few days after the symptoms are gone.

Medications and Supplements

Medications may cause gastritis, which is inflammation of the lining of the stomach. Nausea may come on within minutes or hours after swallowing them.

Well-known medications that cause nausea are narcotics, NSAIDs (nonsteroidal anti-inflammatory drugs), and L-dopa (levodopa). Any combination of sex hormones estrogen, progesterone, and testosterone may also result in nausea. Other types of drugs that may cause nausea and vomiting include antibiotics and antivirals.

Basically, all prescription medications and some over-the-counter drugs and supplements can result in nausea. Always make sure you read the labels on the bottle for instructions for taking them with or without food. This may help reduce the upset. Another important factor to consider is the timing and combination of the doses of the medications prescribed to you. Some of you may want to stop taking medications because you think they are the problem. However, you should always speak with your doctor before stopping or changing any of the medications you take. Your pharmacist is also an expert resource for this information, especially when you are receiving a new drug prescription. It is always a good idea to read the paperwork that comes with the medications from your pharmacy. Hold onto those documents for a while to refer to if needed.

Alcohol

Drinking alcohol in excess can certainly end up causing nausea. Too much alcohol can cause the lining of your stomach to become inflamed, resulting in gastritis. Other symptoms may include headache, dry mouth, and fatigue. This problem usually resolves itself, and of course, it can be avoided.

If you are going to drink alcoholic beverages, a few things can be done to try to prevent becoming nauseated and possibly vomiting. Make sure you have food in your stomach to slow the absorption of alcohol. Be aware of how the medications you take may interact with alcohol. Some medications require you do not drink alcoholic beverages while taking them. If severe vomiting persists after you had excess alcohol, seek medical attention, as alcohol poisoning or overdose can result in seizures, coma, and death.

Food Poisoning

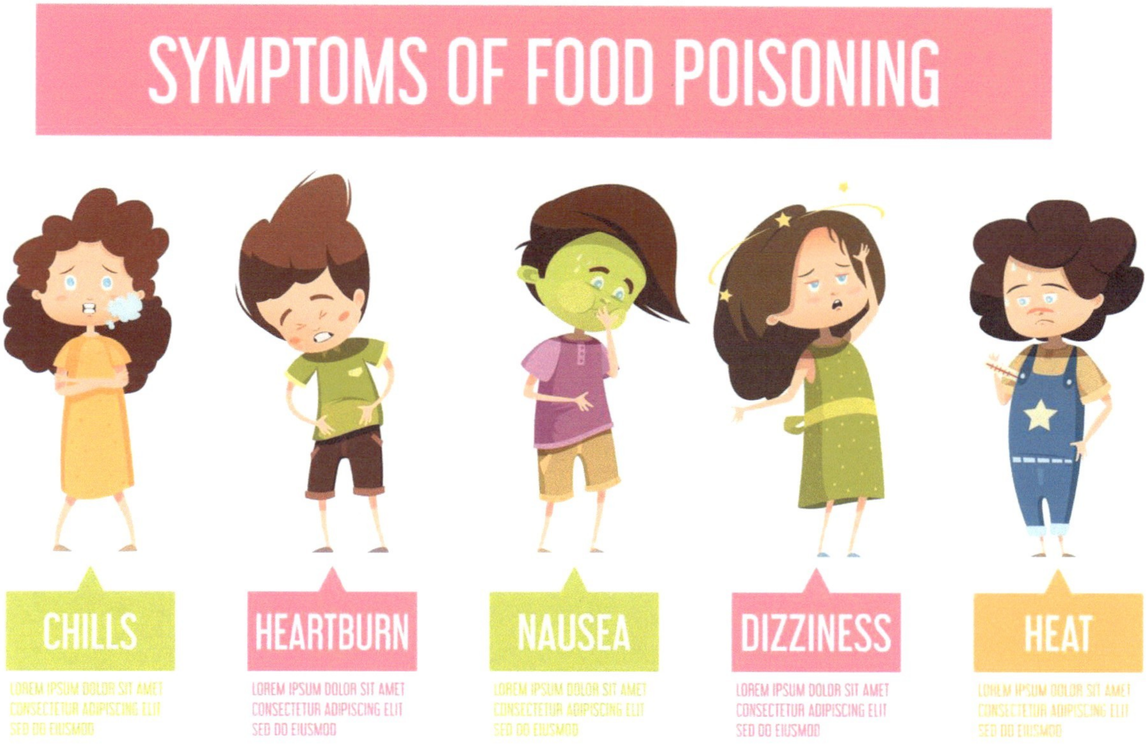

Figure 3.1: Food poisoning symptoms

Although it is a liberally used term by the public, food poisoning is uncommon. However, when it does occur, there are reports in the media, and the source of the poisoning is disclosed to decrease further contamination throughout the community. If the source of the bacteria is in a food sold in a grocery store, you will hear about recalls of those certain items.

The U.S. Food and Drug Administration at www.fda.gov states the following: "While the American food supply is among the safest in the world, the Federal government estimates that there are about 48 million cases of food-borne illness annually—the equivalent of sickening 1 in 6 Americans each year. And each year these illnesses result in an estimated 128,000 hospitalizations and 3,000 deaths."

Make sure your produce is fresh and washed well prior to using. Look at dates on prepared food, and refrigerate everything that calls for it.

Some types of food poisoning cause nausea and vomiting, stomach cramps, and diarrhea temporarily, while others can be lethal, especially to young children and the elderly. Therefore, it is very important that you go to the emergency department of your local hospital or see your physician if your symptoms worsen instead of getting better.

Three common bacteria that cause food poisoning are E. coli, salmonella, and listeria. Less common illnesses that can be transferred from food or food handling are botulism and infections from campylobacter and shigella.

Headaches and Other Neurological Conditions

A migraine headache is very different from a bad headache. Some call them *sick* headaches because of the frequent association with nausea and vomiting. Additional symptoms can include extreme sensitivity to light and sound, along with pulsating pain on one or both sides of the head. In essence, you experience an overall unpleasant hypersensitivity to stimuli. Some people have visual symptoms such as seeing spots or stripes that are referred to as auras.

Migraine headache pain results from signals interacting among your brain, blood vessels, and surrounding nerves. During a headache, specific nerves of the blood vessels are activated and send pain signals to the brain. It's not clear why these signals are activated in the first place. Triggers for migraines include emotional stress, changing weather conditions, fluorescent light, exhaustion, food allergies, and hormonal changes.

New and severe headaches with changes in vision may also need an emergency evaluation to exclude many things, such as meningitis, stroke, hypertension, autonomic nervous system dysfunction, and various forms of seizure disorders. All of these can cause nausea and vomiting and need to be investigated.

Motion Sickness

Almost everyone has had motion sickness at one time or another. It could have been while riding on a boat (seasickness) or going around tight mountain curves (car sickness). This cause of nausea and vomiting is usually sudden in onset. Most of you know if motion causes you nausea and discomfort and avoid situations that may bring this on. Regarding car sickness, some people find it more comfortable to sit in the front seat instead of the rear of the car. There are various devices to stimulate Chinese acupuncture pressure points that can be soothing and help to reduce nausea. Also, a scopolamine patch can be beneficial if traveling by plane or ship. Dramamine™ is also a standby if motion induced nausea is a repeating discomfort for you.

Pregnancy

Approximately 80 percent of women experience nausea and vomiting in the first three to four months of pregnancy. We usually refer to this as morning sickness. Those of you who have experienced it with light-headedness or exhaustion the entire day must wonder why they call it morning sickness. Nausea and vomiting can easily cause a loss of appetite. Many women worry that this will harm their babies. Mild morning sickness is generally not harmful.

Women who experience morning sickness well beyond the first three to four months of their pregnancies should discuss this with their doctor. It is possible that if you continue to be nauseated and vomit past that stage in your pregnancy you may be experiencing hyperemesis gravidarum. If you are also experiencing dehydration, headaches, low blood pressure, and weight loss, you should immediately seek medical help. We hope the three-step diet described in chapter 5 will help with your nausea, but you should review the diet with your doctor to be sure it is appropriate for you, as it is a low-fat and low-fiber diet.

Pain

If you are in an accident and break a bone, have a head injury, or have immense internal pain, you feel acute pain. Initially, you may not even feel the pain, as your body is in shock to protect you. When such an event occurs, your sensory nerves respond and immediately send signals to the spinal cord that something is wrong. Your spinal cord sends messages straight to the brain, and there the decision is made on how your body will respond. Your nervous systems go into overdrive. Your brain will then determine whether to evoke tears, raise your heart rate, or produce adrenaline, endorphins, or other reactions, including nausea and vomiting – or all the above.

Indigestion

Indigestion—also called an upset stomach—is a general term that describes mild discomfort in your upper abdomen. Indigestion is not a disease but rather a term used by patients and advertisers to describe symptoms. These symptoms are abdominal discomfort or pain, fullness, and nausea soon after you start eating or after you finish eating. Indigestion is common, yet each person may experience it in a different way. Most all of us self-treat this feeling with over-the-counter products. However, this discomfort can be a symptom of another digestive disease. Therefore, it is important to understand how often you are feeling indigestion and if it is getting worse over time. The over-the-counter remedies may work for immediate relief, but they may not be the ultimate cure. If symptoms recur over time, your indigestion may be caused by an underlying medical disease.

Gastroesophageal Reflux Disease (GERD)

GERD is reflux of stomach acid into the esophagus that causes a burning sensation in the middle of the chest—i.e., heartburn. GERD is present if you have heartburn two or more times a week. The stomach acid travels back up into your esophagus through the lower esophageal sphincter, causing the burning sensation. Around 20 percent of Americans have GERD. Most who suffer from this disease self-treat for a time with antacids. Again, it is important to track the frequency of your heartburn episodes and try to adjust your diet. You may want to limit common offending foods, such as tomato sauces, fruit juices, and chocolate. GERD can also present as a sore throat, a dry cough, nausea, and even chest pain sometimes thought to be a heart problem, which is where the term *heartburn* comes from. If any of these symptoms persist, it is important to see your doctor. Frequent heartburn can damage the esophagus. *It should be noted that anytime you or someone you care for experiences acute chest pain that is not familiar, call 911 immediately.*

APPENDICITIS SYMPTOMS

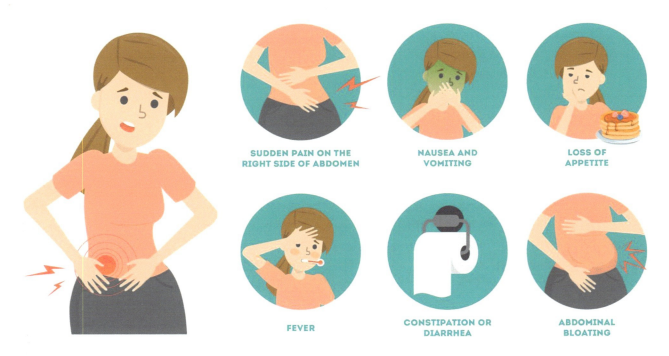

SUDDEN PAIN ON THE
RIGHT SIDE OF ABDOMEN

NAUSEA AND
VOMITING

LOSS OF
APPETITE

FEVER

CONSTIPATION OR
DIARRHEA

ABDOMINAL
BLOATING

Figure 3.2: Appendicitis symptoms

Appendicitis occurs when mucus, a foreign object, or stool blocks the opening between the appendix and the cecum. The blockage causes irritation, inflammation, and possibly infection. Pain in your lower-right abdomen is a sign of inflammation and/or infection. You may experience the symptoms in figure 3.2.

Just as in most other causes of nausea and vomiting, appendicitis can be acute or chronic. In the United States, appendicitis is the most common cause of abdominal pain resulting in surgery. More than 5 percent of Americans experience appendicitis. If left untreated, it is possible your appendix could burst, causing bacteria to spill into your abdominal cavity. This is called bacterial peritonitis and is serious and sometimes fatal.

Gallbladder Disease

The gallbladder, attached to the liver, is a pear-shaped organ that stores bile produced by liver and aids in fat digestion. Over time, stones of cholesterol, bilirubin, and calcium can form in the gallbladder. They can be as small as a grain of sand or as large as a golf ball. Gallstones may cause pain during a gallbladder attack. While not all gallstones cause symptoms, they can lead to inflammation of the gallbladder—i.e., cholecystitis. Bile salts and crystals can also irritate the gallbladder and clog the ducts, resulting in similar symptoms. Inflammation can cause symptoms without gallstones present.

Pain in the upper-right side of your abdomen may indicate a gallbladder attack. Pain usually increases and decreases during the one to five hours following a meal. The pain can radiate into your back and even reach your shoulder. The intake of fatty foods often triggers the pain. After one painful attack, it may be a day, a week, or months before the next attack occurs. Radiographic tests can diagnose the presence of gallstones and inflammation. Blood test can establish the presence of increased liver injury or pancreatic enzymes, which may indicate a blockage of the common bile duct caused by the passage of a gallstone.

The sudden severe pain of a gallbladder attack can require immediate hospitalization for evaluation and treatment of gallbladder diseases. Other symptoms you may notice prior to the pain are indigestion, nausea, vomiting, and fever.

Peptic Ulcer Disease (PUD)

PUD is open sores or ulcers in the lining of the stomach and duodenum. The stomach lining is normally protected from corrosive acid juices by a thick layer of mucus. PUD may be caused by an infection from a microorganism called Helicobacter pylori (H. pylori). Other causes are alcohol and use of NSAIDs.

Symptoms of PUD include painful burning sensations in the upper-mid abdomen, nausea, vomiting, and bloating. In a serious case of peptic ulcer disease, vomiting blood, severe pain in the upper abdomen, and tarry-black stools require immediate attention in the emergency department.

Depending on the underlying cause of the ulcers, you may be prescribed antibiotics for H. pylori or drugs that reduce acid, like H_2 receptor blockers, or proton pump inhibitors, like Nexium™.

Anesthesia

If you have had surgery, you may have experienced nausea and vomiting after you awakened. Hopefully, your surgery was not too invasive and could be performed without too much pain. If you have a large incision, vomiting itself may be very painful. Postsurgical nausea and vomiting can be caused by the anesthesia drugs, pain medications, the pain itself, or a combination of all.

As we transition into a world where more noninvasive surgeries are performed, less anesthesia and fewer pain medications will be required. This means patients are less likely to have nausea and vomiting after surgery. Follow your doctor's orders for how best to recuperate.

Chemotherapy

Chemotherapy is drug treatment that uses powerful chemicals to kill fast-growing cells in your body. It is used to treat cancer because cancer cells grow and multiply much quicker than normal cells. Many different chemotherapy drugs are available. While an effective treatment for many types of cancer, chemotherapy also carries a risk of side effects. Nausea and vomiting are two of these side effects.

Follow your doctor's orders for how to manage your nausea at home. Also, review the three-step nausea and vomiting diet described below with your cancer doctor, as it may help you hydrate and nourish yourself if nausea is not completely helped with medications.

Radiation Therapy

High doses of radiation therapy are used to destroy cancer cells. Side effects come from damage to healthy cells and tissues near the treatment area. Everyone's experience with radiation therapy is different. Side effects vary from person to person, even when given the same type of treatment.

Much research has been done in recent years that has made radiation therapy more precise. This has reduced side effects compared to radiation techniques used in the past. The part of your body being treated may elicit different side effects. Reactions to the radiation therapy often start during the second or third week, and they may last for several weeks after the final treatment. Some side effects may be long term. Talk with your treatment team about what to expect and review the three-step diet with your radiation therapy doctors if your nausea is not completely controlled.

Causes of Chronic Nausea and Vomiting

Chronic illnesses are distinguished from the acute in that they continue for weeks, months, or sometimes years. In this section, gastrointestinal diseases and disorders that are associated with chronic nausea and vomiting are reviewed.

Obstructions of the Gastrointestinal Tract

Over time, blockage due to benign or malignant lesions in the GI tract (in contrast to sudden or acute blockages) can result in nausea and vomiting. In this situation, abdominal pain often becomes a dominant symptom. The specific location of your pain is important to articulate because it will lead your physician to the right organ causing the pain. This can be difficult and frustrating because there are so many different organs within the abdomen. For example, if the pylorus of the stomach is obstructed, then the stomach cannot empty. Your food and drink have nowhere to go except backward. Therefore, nausea and vomiting occur. There is usually severe, cramping pain in the upper abdomen before the vomiting occurs. Obstructions of the duodenum, gallbladder, small intestine, and colon may also cause nausea and vomiting and are usually accompanied by abdominal pain.

Gastrointestinal Cancers

These cancers affect the gastrointestinal tract and organs within the digestive system, including the esophagus, stomach, small intestine, pancreas, liver, gallbladder, colon, appendix, and rectum. Each cancer is often associated with some degree of nausea and vomiting in addition to other symptoms from the involved organ itself.

Pancreatitis

Pancreatitis is the most common pancreatic disorder and is dangerous. Symptoms typically come on suddenly and are characterized by abdominal pain, nausea, and vomiting. Once thought to be uncommon, the incidence of pancreatitis has been on an upward trend in the last twenty years. It is believed to be related to increased rates of obesity and gallstones. Acute pancreatitis appears suddenly and lasts for days. Mild cases of acute pancreatitis usually regress without any treatment, but severe cases can cause life-threatening complications.

Chronic pancreatitis is a less common form of pancreatitis that occurs over many months or years and is loaded with potentially severe complications, including pancreatic abscesses, cysts, and cancer. The main preventable causes of pancreatitis in adults are alcoholism, smoking, and obesity. Other causes include gallstones, cystic fibrosis, very high triglycerides, and infections. Nausea and vomiting can be associated with acute and chronic pancreatitis.

Surgical Procedures on the Stomach

If a patient's symptoms are due to stomach diseases and continue to a chronic degree without resolution after medical treatments, surgery may become necessary. After various surgical procedures are performed on the stomach, the normal stomach function can be severely affected, and chronic nausea and vomiting may develop. Several surgical operations are described below:

- A *vagotomy* is a procedure that severs the vagus nerve and is performed for severe nonhealing ulcer disease. The vagus nerve is one of twelve cranial nerves. The vagus nerve runs from your brain throughout most of the gastrointestinal tract, as well as heart and lungs. This nerve is part of the parasympathetic nervous system. The vagus controls functions of the heart, lungs, and GI tract. It also controls secretions from mucous membranes. When the vagus nerve is cut, the stomach produces much fewer contractions and less acid secretion. The decrease in contractions of the stomach may result in gastroparesis, a paralyzed stomach.
- An *antrectomy* is a procedure that removes the antrum of the stomach and is usually performed to treat nonhealing ulcers or cancers of that part of the stomach. Proper milling of food and gastric emptying is reduced. Gastroparesis is possible.
- A *pyloroplasty* is cutting the pyloric sphincter to loosen the pressure created by the muscle of the sphincter. The pylorus helps to regulate stomach emptying. In some people, it is too tight and contributes to delayed gastric emptying and nausea.
- A *fundoplication* is performed for heartburn that is unresponsive to medical treatment. The top part of the stomach, the fundus, is wrapped around the lowest part of the esophagus to help prevent acid reflux. This surgery deforms the part of the stomach that normally relaxes to receive food. Thus, after the operation, people may feel excessively full after they eat, and the antrum may not function properly to mix and empty food.

A Roux-en-Y is another type of gastric operation that is performed when the antrum of the stomach must be removed. This procedure divides the fundus of the stomach from the rest of the stomach, and the remaining pouch is then connected to the small intestine. There is a risk of nausea and vomiting because of the reduced size of the fundus and its ability to empty food. The Roux-en-Y operation or the sleeve gastrectomy are also used to treat morbid obesity, as they dramatically reduce the size of the stomach and result in weight loss.

Diseases of the Endocrine System

There are many diseases of the endocrine system that may affect stomach function. The pancreas islet cells, the adrenal glands, and the thyroid gland are endocrine system glands most often associated with digestion. Common endocrine disorders are diabetes mellitus, adrenal insufficiency, hypothyroidism, and hyperthyroidism.

Diabetes mellitus is the sustained abnormal increase in blood sugar due to decreased insulin secretion (type 1) or insulin resistance (type 2). Someone who suffers with diabetes may develop nausea and vomiting because of abnormal stomach pacemaker function and decreased muscle contractions of the stomach or gastroparesis. Some autonomic nervous system (ANS) abnormalities may also occur, particularly if the glucose levels remain high in your blood over many years.

The adrenal glands, which lie on top of each kidney, secrete a hormone called cortisol. These glands help maintain the proper glucose and electrolyte levels in the body. When you feel stress, they release cortisol. Additionally, cortisol supports basic metabolism. Nausea and vomiting are common symptoms of low cortisol levels due to adrenal gland insufficiency.

Stomach and gastrointestinal contractions are also decreased by hypothyroidism. For some, nausea and vomiting may be the symptoms that present first, and the thyroid disorder is discovered secondarily. Excess thyroid hormone secretion, or hyperthyroidism, may also cause nausea and weight loss.

Medications

As mentioned, medications can also be a cause of chronic nausea. Each medication and the combination of medications you are taking should be reviewed with your physician and/or pharmacist for potential contribution to your nausea symptoms. Keeping your medication list current and accurate in your medical record is your responsibility and of great importance. It would be a good idea to have a list of them and their dosages in your wallet.

Eating Disorders

An eating disorder is a serious psychiatric diagnosis in which limiting eating, increasing exercise, and reducing body weight are an obsession to an unhealthy extent. The person with anorexia nervosa, most often a girl or young woman, initially begins dieting to lose weight. Over time, the weight loss becomes a mechanism of mastery and control. The drive to become thinner is thought to be secondary to concerns about control and fears relating to one's body. The individual continues the endless cycle of restrictive eating. Some patients with anorexia nervosa also have gastroparesis. Often the person can be close to starvation, and death is possible.

Bulimia is also a serious psychiatric diagnosis that occurs chiefly in females. It is characterized by compulsive overeating usually followed by self-induced vomiting, laxative, or diuretic abuse. Bulimia is often accompanied by guilt and depression.

Digestive diseases and disorders that cause nausea and vomiting may seem to look like an eating disorder to others. In caring for and loving someone, it is important not to jump to a quick conclusion about a diagnosis. If someone is experiencing nausea and vomiting from any gastrointestinal reason, it is natural for them to limit their food choices and consumption.

While your nausea and vomiting symptoms are being thoroughly evaluated, it may be beneficial for you or the one you care for to consult with a psychologist or psychiatrist. These consultations are helpful to exclude an eating disorder.

Central Nervous System Diseases

Because not all causes of nausea and vomiting are due to gastrointestinal disorders, it is important to explore problems in other systems of your body. Many central nervous system (CNS) diseases are associated with nausea and vomiting. Symptoms you need to connect and communicate include a headache; light-headedness; changes in hearing, vision, or balance; ringing in the ears; and swallowing problems. Each symptom can give a clue that the main issue is related to the CNS. CNS diseases that cause nausea include Parkinson's disease, orthostatic intolerance, meningitis, seizures, strokes, tumors, and traumatic brain injury (TBI).

Gastric Neuromuscular Disorders

Frequently, the major categories of diseases and disorders that cause nausea and vomiting are excluded by careful medical history, physical examination, and standard blood tests. If standard x-ray studies, endoscopic examination of your stomach, and CAT scans of your abdomen and head are entirely normal, then gastric neuromuscular disorders should be investigated.

The symptoms associated with gastric neuromuscular disorders increase after eating, and many people experience bad digestion or indigestion. The worst symptoms are nausea and vomiting.

If imaging tests and endoscopy are found to be normal, then doctors may diagnose these symptoms as functional dyspepsia. Bad digestion, indigestion, and functional dyspepsia may be very confusing terms to both you and your doctors because they are not specific. These are the symptoms associated with gastric neuromuscular disorders, and diagnostic tests are needed to confirm if you have them.

When talking with your doctor about these symptoms, it will be helpful to you and your doctor if you describe the symptom that bothers you the most. You may describe these sensations as nausea, bloating, or pain, and be sure to point out where the sensation is located on your body. If you are experiencing stomach neuromuscular dysfunction, your symptoms are usually worse after eating. The time after eating is when the neuromuscular activity of the stomach is needed to receive, mill, and empty the meal. Gastric neuromuscular disorders range from the paralyzed stomach to subtle electrical disorders called gastric dysrhythmias. All are described below.

Gastroparesis

Gastroparesis is the most serious of the gastric neuromuscular diseases and can be considered stomach paralysis. The degree of paralysis can range from mild to severe. The more severe the paralysis, the more difficulty the stomach has mixing and emptying solid and liquid foods. Nausea, vomiting, and weight loss may become major problems. Different categories of gastroparesis are known and described below. The specific type of gastroparesis should be diagnosed to allow for appropriate treatment. The different types of gastroparesis are:

- *Idiopathic gastroparesis* refers to the type for which a cause cannot be determined. Idiopathic gastroparesis represents one-third of all the gastroparesis patients. Many patients report a history of an acute, severe viral illness three to six months prior to the beginning of their continual nausea symptoms. It is likely that the virus injured stomach nerves or pacemaker cells called the interstitial cells of Cajal (ICC). These patients can be diagnosed as probable post-viral gastroparesis. In other patients, chronic symptoms of gastroparesis followed exposure to food poisoning, antibiotic, or anesthetic drugs. In some cases, there are simply no clues to the cause. The process that resulted in gastroparesis may have been due to a degenerative or inflammatory disorder that affected the nerve, muscle, or pacemaker cells of the stomach. Almost 25 percent of patients with gastroparesis have normal pacemaker cells and often have pyloric dysfunction that can be treated.

- *Diabetic gastroparesis* symptoms may range from indigestion to severe nausea and vomiting. In January 2022, the CDC estimated 37.3 million Americans have been diagnosed with diabetes. That is equivalent to one in nine Americans. Diabetic gastroparesis affects about 50 percent of people with type 1 and 30 percent of people type 2 diabetes mellitus. These patients have usually had diabetes for ten or more years. Gastroparesis related to diabetes does not usually resolve completely, but better glucose control may help. For diabetic patients with chaotic, hard-to-control blood glucose levels along with nausea and vomiting, the diagnosis of gastroparesis should be suspected. The treatment of diabetic gastroparesis includes proper insulin therapy, dietary counseling, glucose control, and antinausea drugs. Drug therapies to stimulate stomach emptying and/or help stomach electrical rhythm become normal are also used.

- *Postsurgical gastroparesis* should not be a difficult diagnosis to make. It should be suspected in any patient who has had previous stomach operations such as a vagotomy or operations that involve the fundus or antrum of the stomach. Gastroparesis related to surgical operations is difficult to treat because the anatomy of the stomach has been radically changed. Thus, decisions to proceed with stomach operations need to be made after much contemplation, education, and discussion with your doctor.

- *Obstructive gastroparesis* causes slow stomach emptying due to spasm or muscle dysfunction of the pylorus. In some cases, a fixed lesion like an ulcer or cancer at the pylorus is found as the cause of slow gastric emptying and gastroparesis. These patients with an ulcer or cancer at the pylorus are treated with dilation of the stricture at endoscopy if it is benign and a surgical operation if it is cancer. In most patients with gastroparesis and three cycles per minute gastric myoelectric activity, the symptoms are improved by endoscopic treatments of the pylorus with Botox or balloon dilation.

- *Ischemic gastroparesis* is a rare disease but an important diagnosis to make. Ischemic simply means a lack of blood flow to a certain organ. Normal stomach nerve, pacemaker, and muscle function depends on normal blood flow to the stomach. The major arteries that provide blood to the stomach are the celiac artery and superior mesenteric artery. If these arteries become narrowed and blood flow is impaired, the stomach cannot function properly, especially after meals. We hear about blocked arteries of the heart but rarely about those to the stomach. Low blood flow to the stomach causes gastroparesis, nausea, and vomiting. If obstructions in the arteries are found, then stents or surgical bypass operations to correct the obstructions in the arteries can be performed.

Gastric Dysrhythmias

The ICC's, mentioned above, are pacemaker cells of the stomach that regulate the frequency and propagation of stomach contractions. Abnormalities in this electrical pacemaker system of the stomach are called gastric dysrhythmias. The normal pacemaker rhythm averages about three cycles per minute (2.5-3.7 cpm). Rhythms that are too fast are called tachygastria (3.7–10 cpm). Rhythms that are too slow are termed bradygastrias (1–2.5 cpm). A combination of the two abnormal rhythms is termed mixed gastric dysrhythmias. Gastric dysrhythmias are associated with nausea and vomiting.

Relaxation or Accommodation Disorders of the Stomach

These disorders are abnormalities in relaxation, or accommodation, of the stomach after ingestion of solid or liquid foods. The fundus, corpus, and antrum fail to relax as food is ingested. As a result, patients feel uncomfortably full after eating a small volume of food. This is called early satiety. There may also be sensations of abdominal discomfort, bloating, and nausea.

In summary, there are many different causes of nausea and vomiting, and fortunately, most of the symptoms are acute in onset, temporary in duration, and resolve on their own. On the other hand, the causes of chronic nausea and vomiting range from common diseases like acid reflux or ulcers and range from gall stones to gastric neuromuscular disorders. When a specific diagnosis can be made more specific therapies can be designed to help you.

In the next chapter, we review what is involved in the search for a specific diagnosis that is driving your symptoms of nausea and vomiting.

for what is ...
to be best in any re...
point of view.

Diagnosis [ˌdaɪəɡ
identifying or det
cause of a diseas
diseases by the ...
for what is thou

CHAPTER 4

Diagnose Me, Please!

There are many factors that go into diagnosing the cause of your nausea and vomiting. You will first want to consider when to seek care from your physician. If you have been nauseated to the point you are unable to eat or drink for twelve hours or your nausea does not improve after using over-the-counter remedies after twenty-four hours, then you need to see a physician. *If you feel your symptoms are an emergency, call 911.*

Is this an emergency?
Emergency attention is needed if you or the one for whom you are caring has:
- severe abdominal pain
- blood in vomit or stool
- severe headache and stiff neck
- dehydration and fainting

Diagnostic Testing

For non-emergency evaluation of nausea and vomiting, you will likely have an appointment with your doctor or medical providers.

After discussion and physical examination by your health care provider, there may be no worrisome findings. Drugs like Phenergan (promethazine), Compazine (prochlorperazine) or Zofran (ondansetron) may be prescribed to decrease your nausea. If you have other symptoms like abdominal pain and your nausea has continued for days or weeks, additional diagnostic tests may be considered to investigate possible causes. There are tests that are the most telling of your overall health and what is going on in your body right at this moment. Common tests that may be ordered to help diagnose the source of your discomfort include blood work and urinalysis. Imaging tests range from ultrasound to various x-ray studies to CAT scans to MRI. A referral for endoscopy may be made.

Blood Work

Most likely one of the first tests to be ordered is blood work. A phlebotomist will be the one to draw blood from your arm. Blood tests include the following:
- *Complete blood count (CBC)* This is a routine test that measures levels of different components in your blood: white cells, red cells, hemoglobin, hematocrit, and platelets.

- *Basic metabolic panel (BMP)* A basic metabolic panel checks for levels of certain compounds in the blood, such as calcium, glucose, sodium, potassium, carbon dioxide, chloride, blood urea, nitrogen (BUN), and creatinine.
- *Complete metabolic panel (CMP)* This test combines the BMP and additional blood levels: alkaline phosphatase, alanine aminotransferase, aspartate aminotransferase, bilirubin, total protein, and albumin.
- *Lipid panel* This test checks levels of cholesterol. There are two types: high-density lipoprotein (HDL) and low-density lipoprotein (LDL).
- *Thyroid panel* Thyroid hormones regulate your metabolism, heart rate, and temperature. This panel measures thyroid stimulating hormone, T3, T4Cortisol, and C-reactive protein.

Urinalysis

Your doctor may order a sample of your urine that will be examined in the lab. The urinalysis is done to screen for urinary tract infections, kidney disorders, liver problems, diabetes, and other metabolic disorders. Your urinalysis can also detect any blood in your urine. Many of these diagnoses could contribute to nausea and vomiting.

X-ray

X-ray is a common imaging test that's been used for decades. You can think of x-ray as high energy that can penetrate solid objects. An abdominal x-ray is a plain image of the organs in your abdomen. This x-ray film may help to find the cause of your abdominal pain, nausea, and vomiting. It can sometimes detect kidney stones, an obstruction of the gastrointestinal tract, a perforation in the intestines, or an abdominal tumor.

Barium X-ray

An upper gastrointestinal x-ray with barium is used to diagnose abnormalities such as ulcers, tumors, and polyps. Barium is a white chalky substance mixed with water for you to swallow. It coats the inside of the esophagus, stomach, and intestines. Barium absorbs the x-rays and shows up as white on the film. Normal and abnormal characteristics of the organs of the GI tract can be evaluated especially the stomach, small intestine, and colon.

CAT Scan

CAT (computed axial tomography) scans use a combination of x-rays and computer technology to create images. A CAT scan of the abdomen and pelvis is a diagnostic tool used to help detect diseases of your stomach, small bowel, colon, gallbladder, liver, pancreas, and other internal organs. It is often used to determine the cause of unexplained nausea, vomiting, and pain. CAT scanning is fast, painless, noninvasive, and accurate.

The difference between an x-ray and a CAT scan is minor regarding what you are required to do. However, the ability to diagnose diseases could be significant depending on the source of your symptoms. X-ray images are 2D, while CAT scan images are 3D. The CAT scanning machine rotates and takes various 2D images of your body from multiple angles.

All the cross-sectional images (slices) are combined together to provide a 3D image of your abdominal organs, bones, blood vessels, soft tissue, and skin. CAT scans can therefore detect structural causes of nausea and vomiting, such as obstructions, tumors, or cysts.

Magnetic Resonance Imaging (MRI)

MRI is another diagnostic imaging test that may be ordered to examine your GI tract. An MRI scan is a different technology altogether. An MRI uses powerful magnets and radio waves to create the images. You are not exposed to radiation when you have an MRI scan, unlike a CAT scan or x-ray. The MRI applies a magnetic field, lining up each of the protons in your body. The radio waves are applied in short bursts to these protons relaying a signal the MRI scanner picks up. Then the computer processes this signal and creates a 3D image of the examined body areas. The diagnostic images of a CAT scan are typically taken quicker than an MRI scan. For instance, a CAT scan often takes five minutes or less, while MRIs can take thirty minutes or more. An MRI often does a better job at diagnosing problems in the joints, soft tissues, ligaments, and tendons.

Ultrasound

Ultrasound is another diagnostic imaging test. Sound waves, which the human cannot hear, travel through soft tissue and fluids and bounce, or echo, off surfaces that are denser. This is how an image is captured. If the ultrasound is being performed on your gallbladder, no echoes will bounce back if it is free of gallstones. If there are stones, the density will show up in varying shadows of gray.

Ultrasound is frequently used to examine your gallbladder, liver, kidney, pancreas, and thyroid. If you are experiencing nausea and vomiting and other symptoms while pregnant, ultrasound is safe to use. It is safer than the other imaging methods that use radiation.

Endoscopy

Many patients with unexplained nausea and vomiting and normal results of standard tests are referred to gastroenterologists for consultation. The gastroenterologist may recommend an imaging test called an upper endoscopy. An endoscope is a flexible tube with a light and lens at the tip of it. Patients are sedated and monitored closely during endoscopy. Once the patient is asleep, the endoscope is passed through the mouth into the esophagus to inspect the lining of the esophagus, stomach, and duodenum.

In many patients, endoscopy findings are normal, but symptoms continue. If so, tests of gastric neuromuscular function should be considered next.

Gastric Neuromuscular Function Testing

The gastric neuromuscular activities include coordinated peristaltic contractions that require normal muscles and nerves but also normal pacemaker cells. If there are abnormalities or a depletion of cells, especially pacemaker cells, the stomach becomes dysfunctional and symptoms like nausea and vomiting develop after eating.

To establish diagnoses of gastric neuromuscular disorders, several noninvasive tests are available. One test is used to measure gastric emptying, which is the rate at which a standard test meal empties from your stomach. Another test is used to measure the gastric myoelectrical activity (GMA) of the stomach. Normal 3 cpm GMA is the electrical activity that occurs during three-per-minute contractions of the stomach after meals and reflects the presence of the interstitial cells of Cajal.

Gastric Emptying Tests

To assess the overall muscular work of the stomach, a gastric emptying test is ordered. It is a noninvasive test and requires four hours. Initially, you will eat a meal of Eggbeaters™, toast, and jam. A radioactive isotope and the Eggbeaters™ are cooked to allow the meal to be measured through the imaging camera. They taste perfectly fine! Immediately after you finish the meal, an image is taken of your stomach. The amount of food remaining in your stomach is measured by one-minute scans at one, two, three, and four hours following your meal. During each scan, you will be standing. In the time between scans, you will be relaxing in the waiting room.

Your stomach's rate of emptying is compared with emptying rates in healthy people. If 60 percent of the meal remains in your stomach at two hours and if more than 10 percent remains after four hours, then your diagnosis is gastroparesis. Gastroparesis is a slow or weak stomach that is not strong enough to empty the meal in the normal time limit of the test.

In 15 percent of patients with chronic nausea and vomiting, the stomach empties too fast. If that is the case your diagnosis is dumping syndrome.

The SmartPill™

The SmartPill™ is a capsule that measures the pH, pressure, and temperature in your stomach, small intestine, and colon. After an overnight fast, you will swallow the capsule as you are eating a test meal—a granola-like bar and a small amount of water. The recordings from within the stomach, small intestine, and colon are transmitted to a small receiver worn on a belt or on a lavalier. The gastric emptying time is measured, and a diagnosis of normal emptying, gastroparesis, or dumping syndrome is made. Small bowel and colon transit times are also measured by this test.

Electrogastrography

Electrogastrography is the method of recording gastric myoelectrical activity (GMA) from electrodes positioned on the skin of the upper abdomen over the stomach. The signal is called an electrogastrogram, or EGG. The EGG is like the EKG, which measures the electrical activity of the heart. In a healthy person, ingestion of food causes the stomach to contract at a rate of three cycles per minute (cpm). The cells within your stomach that create this 3 cpm rhythm are ICC's, the pacemaker cells of the stomach and gastrointestinal tract. These pacemaker cells were discovered by and subsequently named after Santiago Ramon y Cajal (1852–1934), a Spanish neuroscientist and the first person of Spanish origin to win a scientific Nobel Prize.

GMA is recorded before and after a test meal called the EGG with water load satiety test. After an overnight fast, you will sit in a comfortable chair in a peaceful environment.

The EGG electrodes are positioned on your abdomen, and you drink water until you are completely full during a five-minute time limit. The EGG test records GMA before and for the thirty minutes after you drink the water.

Hopefully, your test results will show the normal 3 cpm GMA pattern. Your results may show weak 3 cpm GMA and gastric dysrhythmias that are too slow (bradygastrias) or too fast (tachygastrias). These findings may relate to your symptoms and abnormal gastric emptying test results.

Many patients, however, have normal gastric emptying tests but have gastric dysrhythmias. These patients have indigestion or what doctors may call functional dyspepsia.

The type of gastroparesis and functional dyspepsia can be determined based on the EGG and water load satiety test results.

Findings of normal or dysrhythmic EGG recordings together with the gastric emptying test results provide vital information about the stomach electrical activity and capacity or relaxation. The combination of test results may help your doctor design drug or diet therapies for you.

Consultation with a Neurogastroenterologist

Additionally, you and your doctor may discuss seeking a consultation with a gastroenterologist who has a special interest in neuromuscular disorders of the stomach and gastrointestinal tract. As mentioned earlier, these doctors may be considered neurogastroenterologists and may have access to special tests needed to diagnosis gastric neuromuscular disorders. If your symptoms are not getting better and no specific diagnoses are established, you may need to discuss a referral to a specialty center for further evaluation and treatment. The American Neurogastroenterology and Motility Society (ANMS) website lists such centers (see the Resources section).

How are nausea and vomiting treated when specific diagnoses are found? An approach to treatment is reviewed below.

Diet, Drugs, and Device Treatments

Diet

The initial treatment of nausea and vomiting is diet with a goal to maintain hydration and nutrition. The diet approaches outlined in this book will help you do this until a specific cause of your nausea and vomiting is found by your medical providers. Even if a specific cause or several causes are found, you may find drug or device therapies described below do not always control your symptoms. Flares of nausea and vomiting may occur. In chapter 5, we review the *Three Step Diet for Nausea and Vomiting* in detail.

Drugs

Drugs for Nausea and Vomiting

There are many drugs for the symptoms of nausea or vomiting and we will review a few of them.. You have probably heard of them, tried them, or are taking them now to treat your nausea and vomiting. The common drugs are Phenergan, Compazine, and Zofran.

There are drugs for nausea caused by chemotherapy agents that your doctor may use to suppress your nausea. One of these drugs is Marinol (dronabinol), which is modeled on the cannabis molecule. Emend (aprepitant) is another drug for chemotherapy-induced nausea that also helps nausea in some patients with gastroparesis and functional dyspepsia. Other classes of drugs that may help nausea in some patients are Elavil (amitriptyline), an antidepressant drug, and Ativan (lorazepam), an antianxiety medication. These drugs reviewed above are *not* specific drugs that address stomach nerve, muscle, and pacemaker dysfunction.

Drugs for Gastric Neuromuscular Disorders

Unfortunately, there are few drugs specifically designed to treat gastric neuromuscular disorders involving poor gastric relaxation, dysrhythmias, and delayed rates of emptying. That is why diet is the first step in treatment.

The only approved drug for stomach neuromuscular dysfunction is Reglan (metoclopramide). Reglan can increase the rate of gastric emptying and decrease nausea, but it also can cause depression. Long-term use can result in Parkinson's symptoms and tardive dyskinesia.

Erythromycin is an antibiotic, but it stimulates strong contractions in the healthy stomach and increases stomach emptying in patients with gastroparesis. It can cause abdominal pain and increased nausea and vomiting. Motilium (domperidone) is a drug that improves nausea, gastric dysrhythmias, and stomach emptying to some degree. It is not approved by the FDA and must be obtained from the FDA through special applications.

No specific drugs for gastric dysrhythmias or problems with gastric relaxation have been approved by the FDA at this time, although several drugs have been shown to decrease the dysrhythmias, as well as the nausea and indigestion symptoms.

Drugs for Acid Suppression

Many patients with chronic nausea and vomiting are treated with drugs that suppress gastric acid, such as proton pump inhibitors (e.g., Prilosec™). These acid-suppressing drugs do not usually help decrease nausea, although in certain instances gastritis and acid reflux into the esophagus can cause nausea rather than typical burning sensations. In these patients, the acid-suppressing medications do help reduce the nausea. Acid-suppressing drugs are usually ineffective in treating nausea related to gastroparesis and functional dyspepsia because the key problem is not the stomach acid. The key problem is neuromuscular dysfunction of the stomach due to the depletion of gastric pacemaker cells and muscle dysfunction of the stomach.

Devices

Gastric Electrical Stimulation

Gastric electrical stimulation is a treatment for uncontrolled chronic nausea and vomiting due to gastroparesis. The stimulation is provided by a device, Enterra ™, that delivers electrical current through two electrodes that are inserted into the stomach wall. The electrodes are implanted into the muscle wall of your stomach during a laparoscopic operation. The stimulator may be considered if you have not responded to drugs or diet therapies. Almost 75 percent of patients with diabetic gastroparesis have decreased vomiting, and those with idiopathic gastroparesis have somewhat less success. The controller for the stimulator is placed within the abdominal wall. The stimulator is adjusted by programing it through the controller.

Nutritional Support Options

For patients with severe nausea and vomiting who cannot maintain their weight, tubes may be needed to provide access to the stomach or small intestine. A gastrostomy tube is a soft plastic tube that is placed through the skin into the stomach for the purpose of venting the stomach to relieve bloating, fullness, and pain. The tube is also used to infuse small volumes of electrolyte solutions, nutritional liquids, and medications.

Another tube can be placed through the gastrostomy tube into the duodenum and the jejunum to deliver liquid nutrition. These are called GJ-tubes, meaning gastrojejunostomy, because the tubes are positioned in both the stomach and the jejunum. The G-tube may be used for venting the stomach, while the J-tube bypasses the weak and dysrhythmic stomach and liquid nutrition can be infused into the jejunum. A dietician and home health experts are involved to select the best formulas for these jejunal, or enteral, feedings. G- and J-tubes may be placed by gastroenterologists during upper endoscopy or by interventional radiologists.

If the stomach cannot be used at all for feeding, then a feeding tube may be placed directly into the jejunum portion of the small bowel for infusing nutrients. These tubes are usually inserted by surgeons, and the operation is a jejunostomy. Enteral feedings can then be provided through the jejunostomy tube.

Finally, if the J-tube feedings cannot be tolerated, perhaps due to small intestine neuromuscular disorders, then total parenteral nutrition (TPN) may be needed to infuse nutrients directly into large veins in the chest through special catheters. TPN is a last-resort approach to nutritional support because the catheters are prone to infections that can lead to serious total body infections called sepsis.

In summary, treatment of nausea and vomiting requires an accurate diagnosis that may require a wide variety of tests to rule out diseases and discover a specific diagnosis causing the symptoms. An accurate and specific diagnosis defines the disease or diseases that are driving your nausea and vomiting symptoms. If a specific diagnosis can be established, then effective treatments are more likely to be found.

Of course, we all want to be nourished and comforted by eating. But if you are experiencing nausea and vomiting for any reason, then you may be unsure about what you should eat. The foods you chose to eat make a difference in the way you feel. When nausea is present and vomiting is a lurking possibility, then the *Three Step Diet for Nausea and Vomiting*, based on gastric physiology and emptying, can help you choose foods to hydrate, nourish, and comfort your uncomfortable stomach.

At this point in your journey through this book, you appreciate the work that a normal stomach and digestive tract do to receive, mix, empty, and absorb the food you eat. You also understand that when gastric emptying, rhythm, and capacity are impaired, nausea and vomiting can occur. Now, what you should eat is the question. In chapter 5, Dr. Koch describes *Three Step Diet for Nausea and Vomiting* in more detail, and Laura reviews the recipes she created to help hydrate and nourish herself.

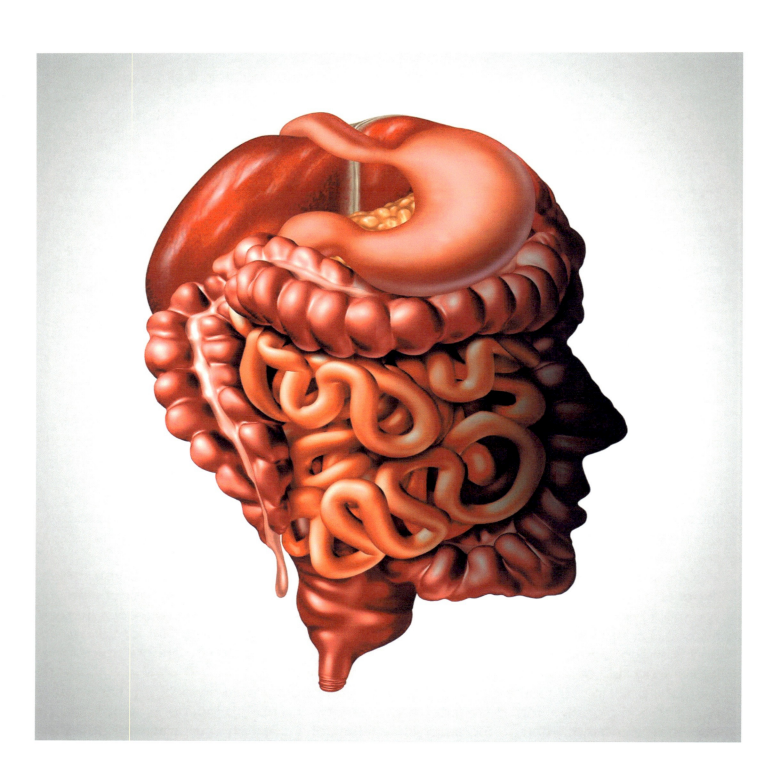

CHAPTER 5

Nourish to Flourish

For patients suffering with nausea and vomiting, thoughtful, careful attention to food selection is very important. Food choices ultimately challenge the mixing, milling, and emptying your stomach must do to sustain your hydration and nutrition.

During many years caring for patients with persistent nausea and vomiting, I learned what kinds of food my patients ate to avoid nausea and especially vomiting. After reading this chapter, you will have this knowledge as well. The dietary approach presented below will allow you to choose foods based on the intensity of your nausea and the frequency of your vomiting throughout the day. With the freedom to choose foods from one of three steps comes control and hope that your choices will provide nourishment, hydration, and even taste good. Many patients have told me the *Three Step Diet for Nausea and Vomiting* helped them avoid trips to the emergency department for intravenous fluids to treat dehydration.

The dietary approach I developed is based on what I learned from patients. I have reviewed the diet in detail with thousands of patients in my clinic during the past thirty years. The *Three Step Diet* has helped many patients stay hydrated, maintain or gain weight, and decrease nausea after eating. I hope you will enjoy reading about and tasting the recipes Laura created to help her hydrate and nourish herself and they will help you feel better, too.

Dr. Koch's Three Step Diet For Nausea and Vomiting

Step 1. Electrolyte Solutions

Diet: Patients with severe nausea and vomiting should sip small volumes of electrolyte replacement liquids such as Gatorade® or broths in order to avoid dehydration. Any liquid to be ingested should have some caloric content. A chewable multiple vitamin is necessary daily.

Goal: For you to get in and keep in ten 4-oz servings over the course of 12-14 hours. 1-2 oz. at a time may be sipped to reach approximately 4 oz. per hour for a total of 40 ounces each 24-hour period.

Avoid: Citrus drinks and highly sweetened drinks. The citric acid within may upset your stomach.

Step 2. Soups and Smoothies

Diet: If electrolyte solutions are tolerated, then you may want to include a variety of soups and smoothies. Peanut butter, cheese, and crackers may be tolerated in small amounts. These foods should be given in at least six divided meals per day. Caramels or other chewy confections may be tried. A chewable multivitamin is necessary daily.

Goal: For you to eat approximately 1,500 calories per day. You will avoid dehydration and get enough calories to maintain your weight and energy level.

Avoid: Heavy milk-based liquids. Avoid fatty liquids as fat will delay emptying of the stomach.

Step 3. Solid Foods

Diet: Starches (carbohydrates) such as noodles, pasta, potatoes and rice are easily mixed and emptied by the stomach. Baked chicken and fish are usually well-tolerated sources of proteins. These should also be ingested in six small meals per day. A chewable vitamin is necessary daily.

Goal: To find a diet of common foods that you find interesting, satisfying, and evoke minimal nausea and vomiting symptoms. As you learn what liquids and solids are tolerated, the variety and number of foods that you can enjoy will increase.

Avoid: Fatty foods which delay gastric emptying, red meats and fresh vegetables which require extensive mixing and milling. Avoid pulpy fibrous foods; they are the most difficult to digest. Including vegetables in a smoothie help your stomach have less work to do while you enjoy their flavor and nutrients.

Table 5.1 Dr. Koch's original Three Step Diet for Nausea and Vomiting

A Deeper Dive into the

Three Step Diet for Nausea and Vomiting

The *Three Step Diet for Nausea and Vomiting* is shown in table 5.1. This is the concise summary of the diet that I go over in detail with patients who have nausea, vomiting and a variety of gastric neuromuscular disorders. I review how each step requires more stomach work to mix and empty and explain that the patient can choose from any step throughout the day depending on the intensity of their nausea. I offer a consultation with one of our dieticians who specializes in advising patients with nausea and vomiting. Most patients want to try out their own selections first. I agree with them because each patient knows his or her stomach the best.

Step 1. Electrolyte Solutions The first Step of the diet emphasizes electrolyte-containing fluids and broths. Step 1 is selected when you or your loved one is having a very bad day with nausea and vomiting episodes. The goal is simply to avoid dehydration. Drinks that provide glucose and electrolytes, such as salt and potassium, are important to sip on to restore volume in the arteries and veins. Athletes understand a very important principle of hydration: water alone *will not correct dehydration*. To rehydrate, electrolytes are required, as well as water. So, on your very bad nausea and vomiting days, try to consume 3 to 4 ounces of electrolyte solution *each hour* to restore and maintain hydration. These little sips of electrolytes and glucose require very little stomach muscular work to be emptied into the small intestine for absorption and hydration. But over the course of ten hours, you will take in 30 to 40 ounces of electrolyte-containing fluids, a volume which should be enough to hydrate you. Fruit juices are *not* recommended because they contain citric acid, which may irritate the esophagus or stomach, especially if you have GERD, and may make your symptoms worse. Also, I suggest you avoid diet drinks or low-sodium bouillon or broth because you need calories and salt on these bad days more than ever. Patients with diabetes need to follow their glucose levels during these bad times of nausea and vomiting.

Step 2. Soups and Smoothies The options in Step 2 can be selected when your nausea is improving, and your vomiting episodes are limited. You and your stomach feel like trying more than broth and electrolyte-containing drinks. Soups such as chicken noodle soup or chicken with rice soup are nutritious liquids and are still relatively easy for the stomach to mix and empty. These soups are salty and contain small amounts of starch. The noodles and rice and small bits of chicken in the soup, consumed slowly in 4- to 6-ounce servings, require minimal work by your stomach. Crackers with small amounts of cheese or peanut butter are also reasonable choices in Step 2. As you see in table 5.1, I also suggest caramels. Patients often ask me why caramels are in Step 2. I usually respond, "Because I like caramels!" But to be serious, I like my patients with nausea to consider caramels because caramels are a food that: 1) require the pleasure of chewing; 2) taste good (to most patients); 3) present very little work for the stomach to accommodate, mix, and empty; 4) provide calories.; and 5) provide an eating experience that is hopefully pleasant and even comforting. This example of the simple caramel represents how food selections should be considered for the patient with nausea and vomiting.

Smoothies with ingredients and flavors that are pleasing to you are another great source of calories, vitamins, and minerals. Smoothies require minimal muscular work by the stomach.

Smoothie ingredients are ready for the stomach to empty because they are already milled by the blender. At this point, smoothies should also be consumed in small volumes four to six times during the day. This is suggested because, for many patients, the stomach has lost some of its ability to relax, which is the neuromuscular function of the stomach to accommodate the amount and type of the food you ingest. So, when you feel full, you need to stop eating because your stomach most likely is at its maximum accommodation. I sometimes advise patients to stop drinking the soup or smoothie when they are 75 percent full so they don't overly challenge the stomach's ability to work. You may also want to try prepackaged protein drinks. Protein drinks have appealing flavors and decrease nausea and gastric dysrhythmias in nausea of pregnancy, motion sickness, and chemotherapy. Adding soy, whey, or other protein powders to your smoothies will add that protein. The goal in Step 2 is to eat in 1,000 to 1,200 calories a day in soups, smoothies, and caramels that taste good and at least maintain your weight. Some patients do very well in terms of hydration, nourishment, and reduced symptoms and continue with Steps 1 and 2.

On the other hand, a patient who was doing well on Step 2 said to me, "Dr. Koch, I just want to be able to chew again." She reminded me about that simple pleasure of mealtime that is lost in the sea of nausea and vomiting. I suggested that she should carefully move to the Step 3 diet choices to find foods she will hopefully tolerate.

Step 3. Solid Foods The options in Step 3 can be selected when nausea is minimal, vomiting episodes are limited, and you are experiencing a little hunger. Solid foods used in this step can be divided into starches, protein, fats, and fibers. Starches require less neuromuscular work compared to proteins, which are easier to mix and empty than fatty foods. Fatty and fried foods delay gastric emptying even in healthy individuals. We get full and stay full much longer when we eat fatty foods compared with starches and proteins. Fibrous foods such as fresh vegetables and fruits have skins and pulp that require the longest time for stomach neuromuscular work.

Thus, Step 3 emphasizes starches such as potatoes, rice, and noodles. Mashed potatoes are the poster food for Step 3. This simple food provides: 1) the pleasure of chewing and swallowing a solid food, 2) limited work for the stomach because potatoes are a starch and are mashed, 3) calories to nourish the body, and 4) the feeling of success that you can tolerate and enjoy a solid food. Rice crispy treats are a food with similar stellar attributes. You will think of many more as you read on and review Laura's recipes below. With some successes with these starches, you will begin to build your Step 3 portfolio of foods that are tasty and provide nourishment to maintain or gain weight.

In Step 3 you should begin to add protein in the form of chicken or turkey breast, chopped or sliced into small pieces, because these foods are relatively easy for the stomach to mix and empty. Fat slows gastric emptying, so fatty and fried foods should be neglected for now. The vegetable fat in peanut butter or olive oil in small amounts is often tolerated. Fibrous foods with skins and pulps are hard for the weak stomach to mix and empty, so they should be avoided.

The *Three Step Diet* is not a complete diet, so it is extremely important to take a gummy multivitamin every day while you select step 1, 2, or 3. The gummy vitamins are great because 1) the pleasure of chewing them can be enjoyed; 2) they are easy to swallow; and 3) the stomach easily accommodates, mixes, and empties them. Horse pills, those large and hard pills that are still manufactured, are difficult to swallow in the best of times and may upset your stomach and even evoke further nausea. See if your doctor can change your horse pills to liquid or gummy formats or crush/cut the horse pills with a pill cutter. Your stomach may feel better with these changes.

Patients described the foods to me that they could keep down *to avoid* nausea but especially to avoid the agonizing, depressing, and embarrassing reflex of unwanted and uncontrollable vomiting. I realized these were the foods that were easier for the normal stomach to mix and empty and therefore would be easier for the weak or dysrhythmic stomach to mix and empty. To make the increasing work of the stomach and increasing dietary selections easier to describe, the *Three Step Diet* came about. My patients understood these concepts that combined their understanding of normal stomach emptying of different foods, their own gastric neuromuscular conditions, the current level of their nausea, and then their choice of foods to drink or eat from Step 1, 2, or 3. This is a process of trial and error. Patients need to go easy, take it slowly initially, and try to advance from Step 1 to Step 2 and then to Step 3.

Laura and I reviewed *Three Step Diet* when she was so nauseated. She understood the stepwise approach to the diet and the condition of her stomach. The diet got her going, but she thought more flavors and more choices were needed within each step. As she mentioned above, she would bring recipes to clinic for sampling, to talk about how she enjoyed them, and ask if they were appropriate for Step 1, 2, or 3. The recipes greatly expand choices in each of the steps. If you want to substitute an ingredient that sounds more appealing you, you should try it. Do everything you can to make your nausea and vomiting decrease. I hope all the recipes below will help you with hydration and nourishment and will comfort your uncomfortable stomach.

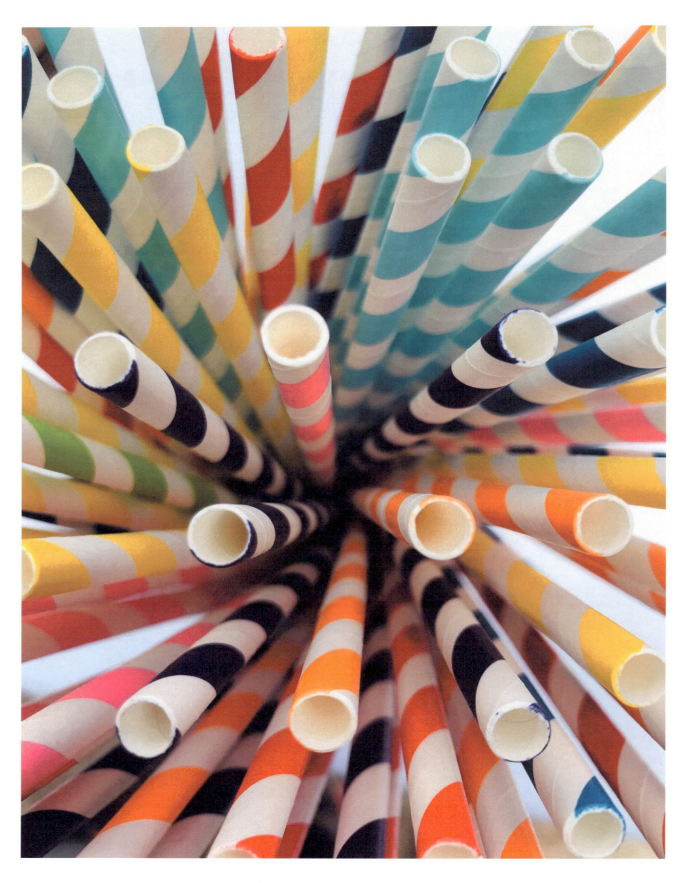

Step 1 Recipes

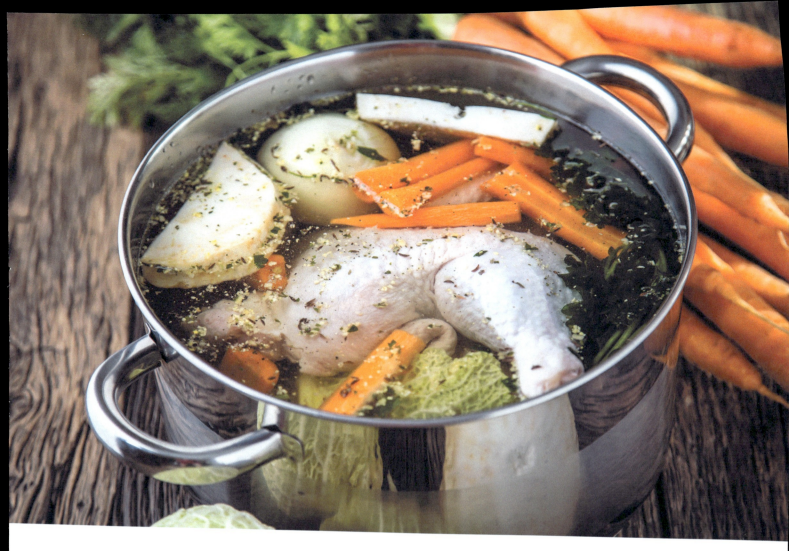

Chicken Stock

1 gallon water (filtered if possible)

1- to 3-pound whole organic chicken (extra bones if available)

1 large onion, peeled and coarsely chopped

2 carrots, peeled and coarsely chopped

3 stalks of celery, coarsely chopped

salt and pepper to taste

2–3 bay leaves

1 bunch fresh parsley (or equivalent of dry parsley)

2–5 tablespoons apple cider vinegar, depending upon size of chicken

Directions

Organic chicken is preferred, as there are more nutrients in the bones and meat. Also, many chickens that are not organic will not produce stock that gels. The ingredients in the gel are good for you. If you are using a whole chicken, make sure you check for a bag in the cavity and remove. If you enjoy those parts, then cook as you like.

Place the whole chicken, vegetables, salt, pepper, and water in large stockpot. Cook over high heat, bringing to a boil.

Reduce heat, cover, and simmer until meat is cooked.

Remove the chicken while the broth continues to simmer and pull the meat from the bones. The chicken meat can be frozen for when you feel better or used immediately in any recipe for your family or friends.

Return the bones to the pot and add the vinegar. Simmer for 6–24 hours.

If you have an organic chicken, you will notice as you stir, the bones begin to become soft. The wonderful apple cider vinegar pulls the nutrients out of the bones for your benefit. Just a few minutes before the chicken stock is ready to remove from the burner, add the mineral-providing parsley.

Strain the pot contents into a large bowl that will easily fit into your refrigerator. Let it cool there overnight.

On the following day, you will find there is a congealed layer on top. This gel is made of good fat and collagen. At this point in your nausea journey, fat and collagen are both helpful additions for your health.

Remove the bowl from the refrigerator and let the broth come to room temperature. If you like, place this broth into covered containers to freeze in small portions. Even ice cube trays can be helpful.

Recipe note: Chicken stock has been a valued remedy for the flu and colds for centuries and still is. Stock also adds to the flavor of other foods. This addition provides protein, salt, and fat that are so desperately needed during a bout with nausea and vomiting. This is so flavorful and a lifesaver at any time.

If you are vegetarian, use all the ingredients in the recipe above except for the chicken. Load it up with your favorite vegetables instead.

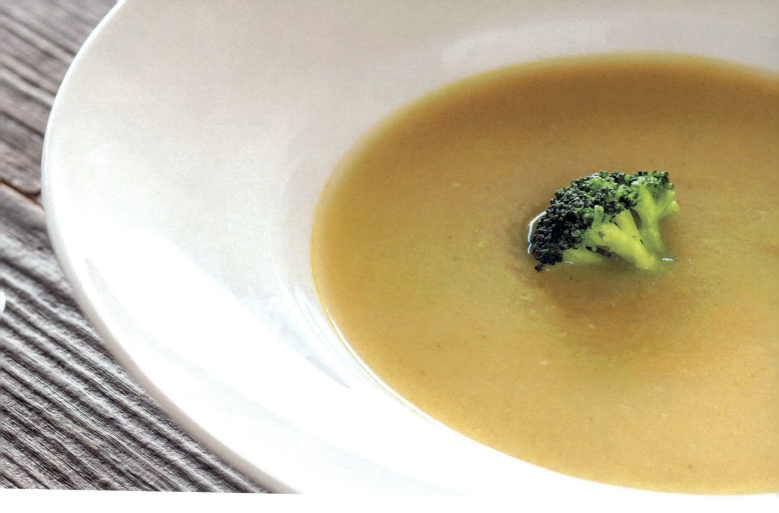

Broccoli and Cheese Broth

3 broccoli florets without stalks, finely chopped

1 small onion, chopped

water to cover

1 cup favorite mild cheese, grated

1/4 stick butter

salt and pepper to taste

Directions

Boil broccoli and onion in water with salt, pepper, and butter.

After 20 minutes, add cheese very slowly while stirring into mixture.

Remove from heat and let mixture cool slightly. Place in blender and puree.

Note: If this puree is too thick for you, strain mixture through cheese cloth to achieve a tasty broth.

I came up with this recipe as I was craving other flavors. It worked for me. Try anything you want to, making sure it is easy for your stomach's work.

Recipe note: Broccoli is a great source of vitamin A. Always purchase fresh green broccoli to ensure the most nutrients available. You end up with amazing flavor and none of the hard-to-digest effects of broccoli. The key is to finely chop the heads. You jump-start digestion by chopping it into small bits. I knew I was on my way to healing after eating this. It was real food and delicious. LD

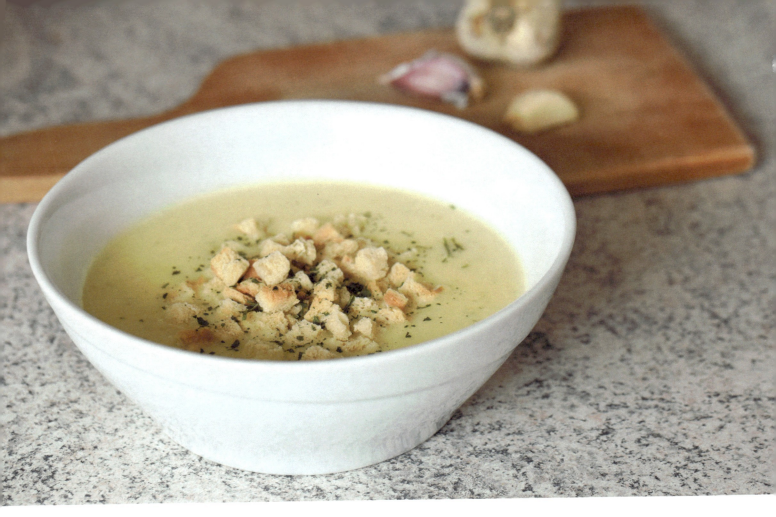

Cauliflower Broth

1 head cauliflower florets
1/4 stick butter
1 bouillon cube (or chicken, beef, or vegetable broth)
salt and pepper to taste

Directions

Place cauliflower florets into a stock pot and add enough water to cover. Add butter, salt, and pepper to taste.

Cook for approximately 20–30 minutes or until tender. You may also substitute riced cauliflower, which is easily found in the frozen food section of your grocer.

Place all ingredients plus bouillon cube or broth in blender to puree.

Recipe note: Cauliflower stimulates your immune system and is rich in vitamin C and potassium. I love the flavor of this soup. It reminds me of my mother packing my lunch in elementary school and including raw cauliflower. That was way before it became popular. She was teaching me good nutrition then. It also makes me laugh to tell my great nieces and nephews that we did not have ranch dressing to dip it in when I was growing up. They are very concerned by that. LD

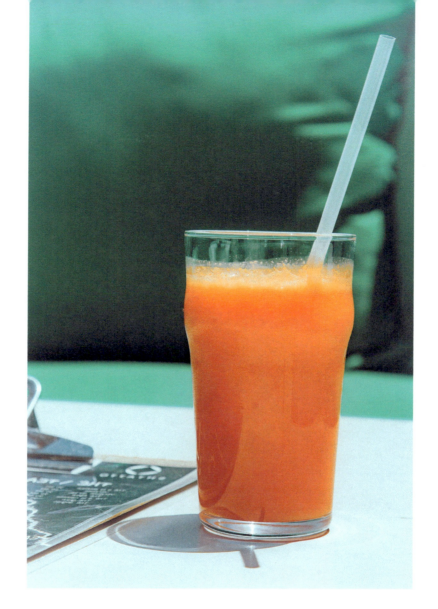

Carrot Broth

3 or 4 large carrots, chopped
sliced fresh ginger or ginger powder to your preferred taste
pinch of salt
water to cover

Directions

Place carrots and ginger in a stock pot and add water to cover.

Cook on high for 15 minutes.

Remove from heat and allow to cool enough to not burn you if it should splatter. Either using an immersion blender or a traditional blender, puree for a sweet, refreshing broth to serve warm or cold.

Recipe note: This receipt is very good for dehydration, as it supplies the liquid to deliver potassium, Vitamins A, C, and E.

My sweet dog, Sadie, would bark her head off every time I cooked this! LD

51

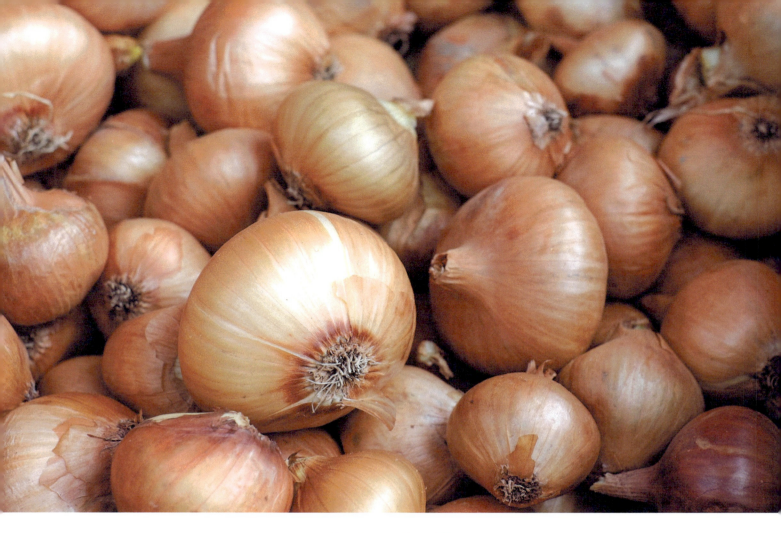

Onion Broth

8 cups water

10 cubes beef bouillon

1 can beef bone broth

6 large onions, finely chopped

3 tablespoons flour

1/4 stick butter

Directions

Combine all ingredients except for flour in large pot and bring to a boil. Simmer for 1 hour. While whisking, add flour for thickening. Cook for 1 more hour.

Run all ingredients through a food processor or blender and press onions out to achieve liquid and to maximize nutrients.

Recipe note: As your stomach will allow, this is a good sauce for pasta or polenta if it is a little thicker.

My mother spoke often of the cleansing and healing properties of onions. She remembered learning this when her father was ill from cancer in the late 1930s. Evidently, my grandmother summoned a healer from the mountains of North Carolina who suggested a diet full of onions would help him in his fight. I am grateful for all I learned about the comfort of nutrition from them. LD

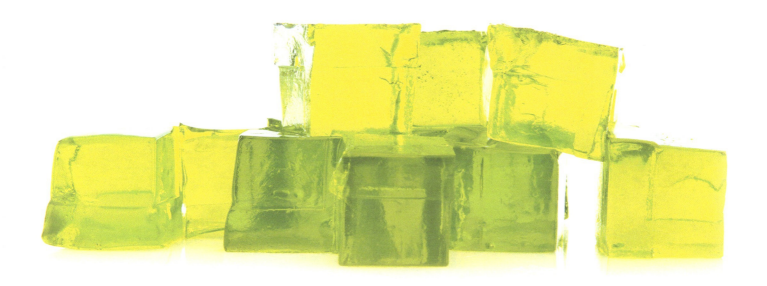

Flavored Gelatin with Electrolyte Drink

small box any flavor gelatin
2 cups electrolyte drink of choice

Directions

Prepare flavored gelatin according to the instructions on the box, replacing the water with your electrolyte drink.

Use any mold you may have on hand for shapes to delight you or those for whom you are caring. Also, mix flavors as you desire.

If you happen to be vegetarian or vegan, replace the flavored gelatin with 4 tablespoons of agar-agar, which is gelatin from sea vegetables. Please also substitute agar-agar in any other recipes with gelatin.

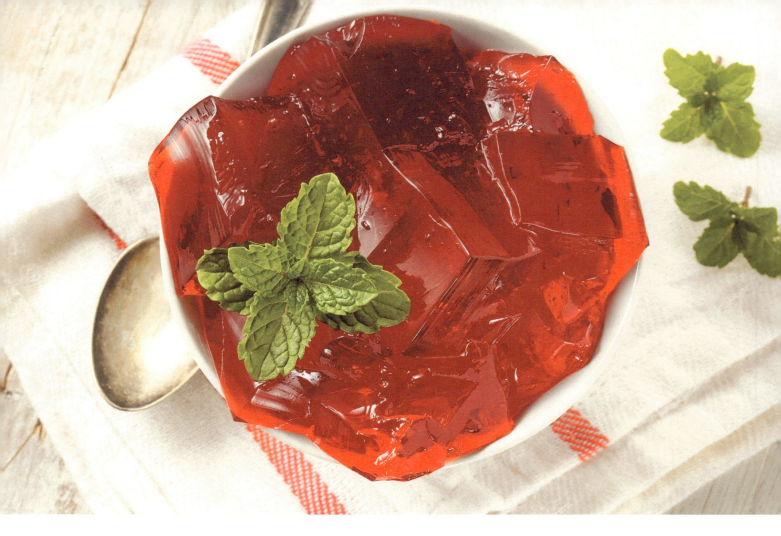

Berry and Applesauce Gelatin Salad

2 cups unsweetened applesauce
1 box cherry gelatin
1 box strawberry gelatin
1 1/2 cups ginger ale

Directions
Poor applesauce into a saucepan and warm over medium heat.
Dissolve flavored gelatin into hot applesauce. Add remaining ingredients and stir well.
Pour mixture into pan and refrigerate until gelatin sets.
Recipe note: Combine any flavors of gelatin that you prefer.
"The beneficial properties of gelatin with food have been studied to a great extent. Gelatin acts first and foremost as an aid in digestion and has been used successfully in the treatment of many intestinal disorders, including hyperacidity, colitis, and Crohn's disease. Although gelatin is by no means a complete protein, it acts as a protein sparer, allowing the body to more fully utilize the complete proteins that are taken in." Sally Fallon, *Nourishing Traditions*, 2001.

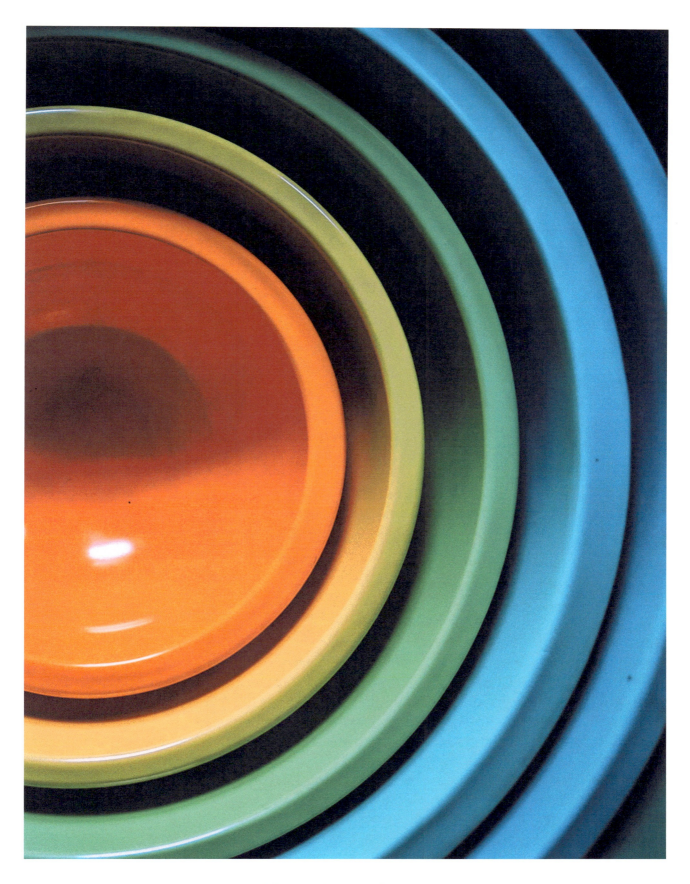

Step 2 Recipes

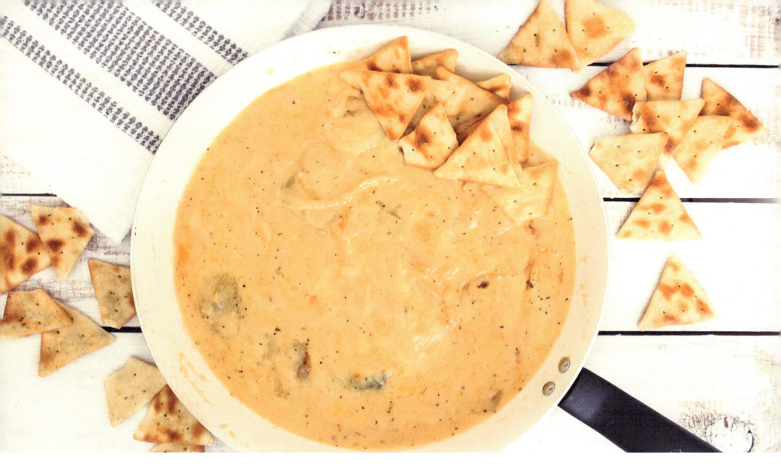

Hummus

1 (15-ounce) can chickpeas, drained and rinsed

1/2 teaspoon baking soda

1/4 cup lemon juice (from 1 1/2 to 2 lemons)

1 medium to large clove garlic, roughly chopped1/2 teaspoon salt

1/2 cup tahini

2–4 tablespoons ice water, more as needed

1/2 teaspoon ground cumin

1 tablespoon extra-virgin olive oil

Directions

Place the chickpeas in a medium saucepan and add the baking soda.

Cover the chickpeas by several inches of water and bring them to a boil over high heat. Continue, while watching, for about 20 minutes, or until the chickpeas are soft.

Drain the chickpeas very well and run cool water over them for about 30 seconds. Set aside.

Meanwhile, in a food processor or high-powered blender, combine the lemon juice, garlic, and salt, preferably mixing for 10 minutes or longer.

Add the tahini to the food processor and blend until the mixture is thick and creamy texture.

With the food processor on, drizzle in 2 tablespoons ice water. Mix until it is smooth, pale, and creamy.

Add the cumin and the drained chickpeas to the food processor. While blending, drizzle in the olive oil.

Blend until the mixture is super smooth, scraping down the sides of the processor as necessary. Blend for about 2 minutes. Add more ice water by the tablespoon if necessary to achieve a super creamy texture. Yummy!

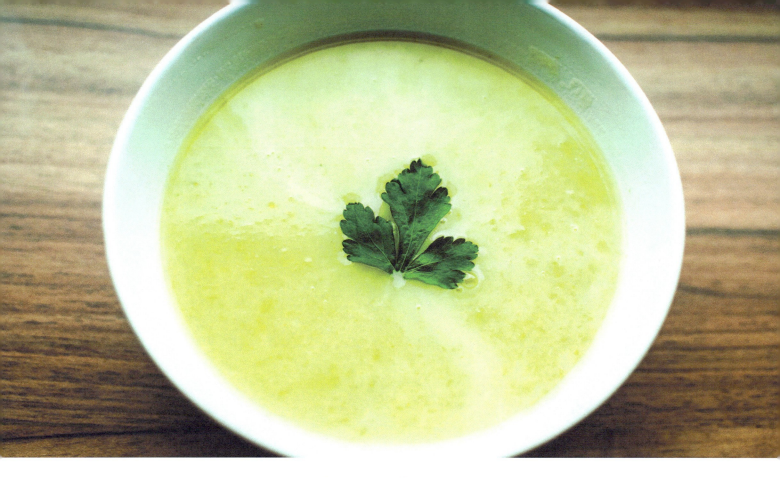

Celery Soup

2 onions, peeled and chopped

3 tablespoons olive oil

1 large head of celery, strings peeled

2 potatoes, peeled and diced

water or favorite broth to cover

salt and pepper to taste

fresh parsley, chopped

Directions

Combine all ingredients in a large pot.

Cook for 1 1/2 hours over medium heat.

Remove from heat and allow to cool slightly.

Place mixture in blender and puree. Strain if necessary for your stomach.

Recipe note: Celery aids in digestion and lowers blood pressure. It is a good source of vitamins A, B, and C, as well as magnesium, iron potassium calcium, sulfur, sodium, phosphorus, and iodine.

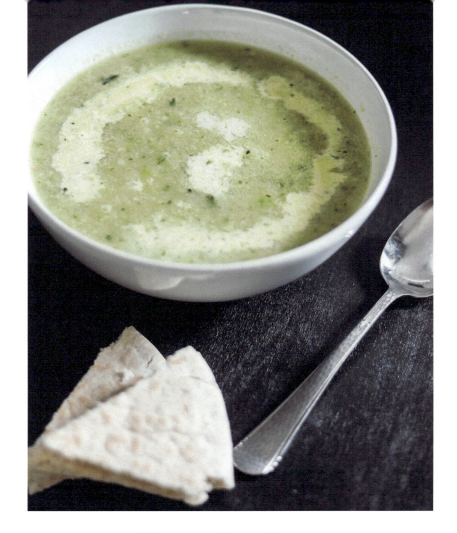

Cucumber Soup

2 tablespoons olive oil
2 onions, diced
1 1/2 quarts chicken broth or stock
2 pounds cucumber, peeled and finely chopped (English cucumbers if the seeds bother you)
salt and pepper to taste

Directions

Cook onions in oil over medium heat for approximately 20 minutes.

Add broth or stock to pan and bring to a boil.

Add cucumber and simmer for 15 minutes.

Remove from heat. Once slightly cool, transfer mixture to blender and puree.

Add salt and pepper to taste.

Recipe note: Cucumber is healing to the stomach and intestinal tract. Both cucumber and onion are blood cleansers. This recipe could be served chilled or hot. Cut a few extra slices of cucumber to place over your eyes if they also need soothing.

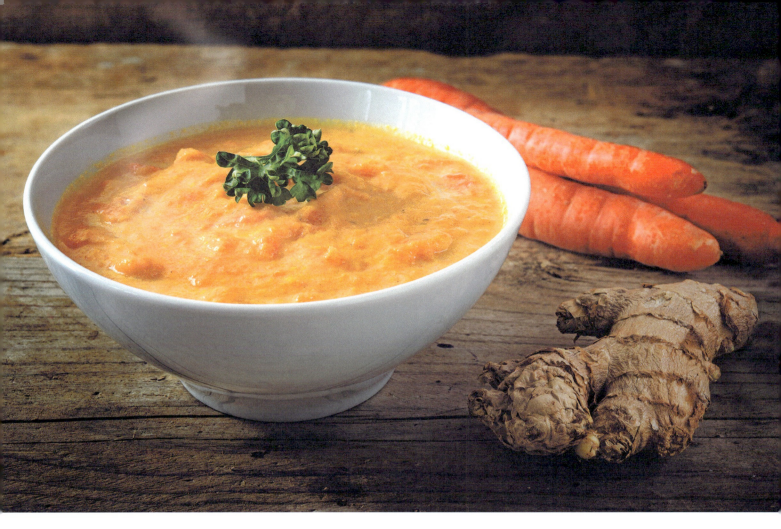

Ginger Carrot Soup

2 tablespoons butter

5 cups chopped carrots

1 1/2 quarts chicken broth or stock

2 tablespoons grated ginger

1 onion, peeled and chopped

1 celery stalk, peeled and chopped

1 medium potato, peeled and chopped

Directions

Melt butter in a sauce pan over medium heat.

Add onion and celery and cook for 10 minutes, stirring occasionally.

Add carrots, potato, ginger, and broth. Bring to a boil.

Reduce heat and cover. Simmer for 20 minutes.

Remove from heat and allow to cool slightly. Place all ingredients into blender and puree.

Recipe note: Ginger aids in digestion and helps decrease nausea symptoms. Carrots are high in beta-carotene, vitamin B complex, calcium, phosphorus, sodium, potassium, and magnesium, all of which help prevent dehydration.

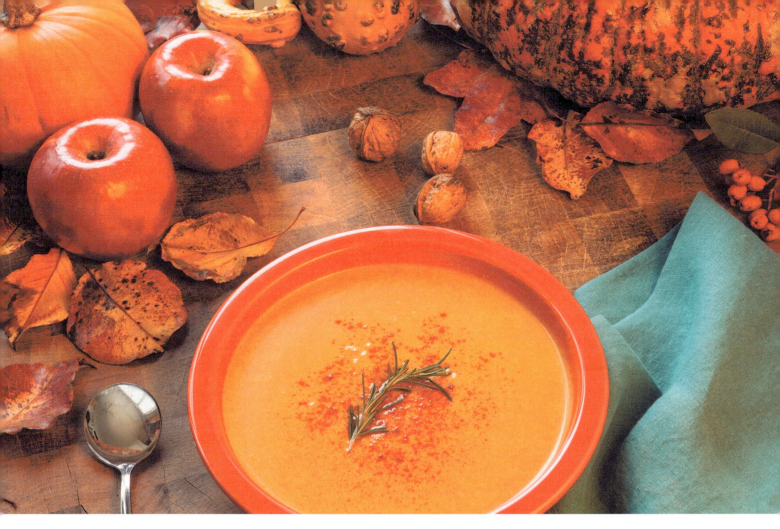

Pumpkin and Apple Soup

4 apples, peeled, cored, and chopped

1 tablespoon butter

1 onion, peeled and chopped

2 cloves garlic, minced

1 (15-ounce) can pumpkin puree

1 quart chicken broth or stock

1 cup water

1 teaspoon salt

Directions

Melt butter in a large saucepan over medium heat.

Add onion and garlic and sauté until soft.

Stir in apples, pumpkin, broth, water, and sugar.

Bring to a boil, stirring often. Cover and reduce heat to simmer. Cook for 25 minutes, stirring occasionally.

Remove from heat and allow to cool slightly. Puree soup in a food processor or blender.

Return soup to saucepan and reheat covered over low heat. You may even enjoy this cold!

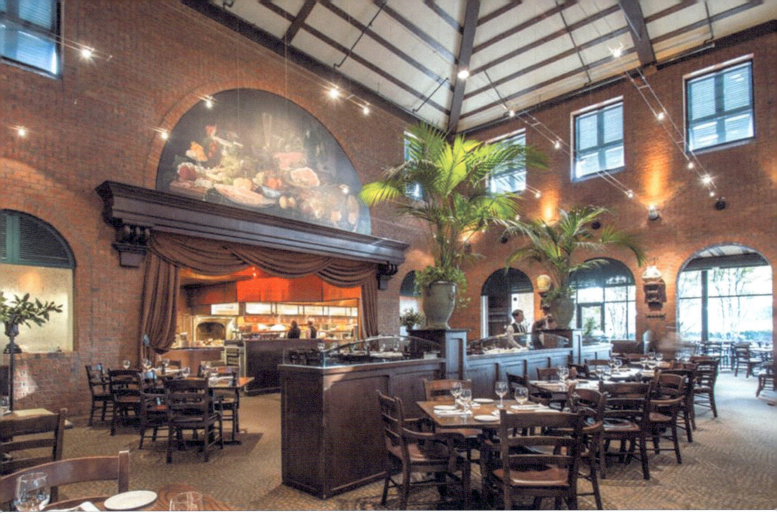

Green Valley Grill Potato Leek Soup

3/4-pound leeks

1 stick unsalted butter

1/2 teaspoon minced garlic

1 1/2 pounds diced Yukon Gold potatoes

3 cups water

2 1/2 cups heavy whipping cream

3/4 teaspoon salt

3/4 teaspoon ground white pepper

fresh chives, chopped for garnish

Directions

Thoroughly clean leeks and remove green stems. Cut white part of leeks in half lengthwise and then in 1/4-inch half-moons.

Melt butter in medium-size sauce pan over medium heat.

Add leeks and garlic and sauté until leeks are soft but not yet browned, about 10 minutes.

Add diced potatoes and water. Bring to a boil and then reduce to a simmer.

Cover partially and simmer 20–25 minutes or until potatoes are thoroughly cooked.

Add cream and bring to a boil.

Remove from heat and let stand until cool. Puree mixture in blender.

Return to pan, warm through, and then season with salt and pepper. Garnish with chopped chives.

Makes: 2 quarts

Disclaimer: This recipe was originally designed for a much larger batch size. This recipe has been reduced but not tested at this scale. Please adjust to your taste and portion size. This recipe is property of Quaintance-Weaver, Inc., and unauthorized commercial use is forbidden.

Recipe note: The Green Valley Grill has fed me several times a week since they opened in 1998. That frequency did not diminish when I was the sickest. GVG is the place I could go, have a social experience, and eat. They make their own delicious chicken broth. As I healed from gastroparesis, they continued to accommodate me by adding some pasta in the broth. Beyond their menu, the environment itself was very healing. It is a transporting space within the O. Henry Hotel in Greensboro, North Carolina, with the most welcoming staff in the industry. A destination for sure! Thank you, Dennis and Nancy Quaintance and Martin Hunt for feeding my body, mind, and soul and for all you do for our community! LD

www.greenvalleygrill.com

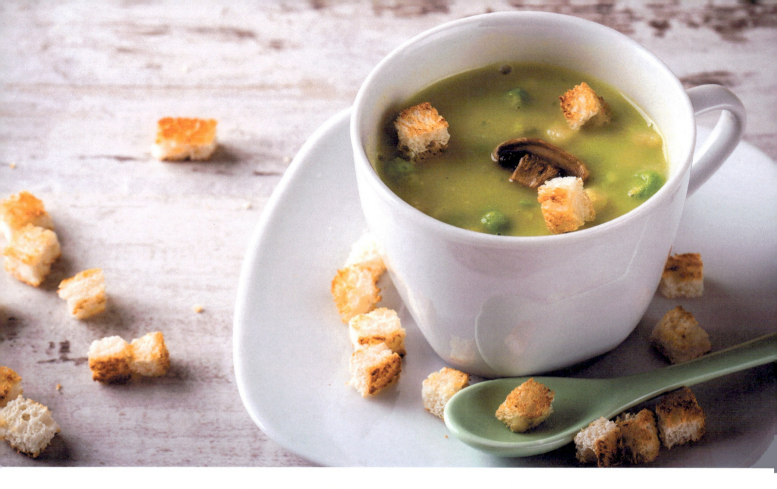

Pea and Mushroom Soup

2 cans small green peas
1 can cream of mushroom soup
1 can water
1 tablespoon olive oil
salt and pepper to taste

Directions

Combine all ingredients in a large pot and cook for approximately 30 minutes.

Place cooled mixture in blender to puree.

Recipe note: Peas contain carotene and vitamin C and help to control blood sugar and lower blood pressure.

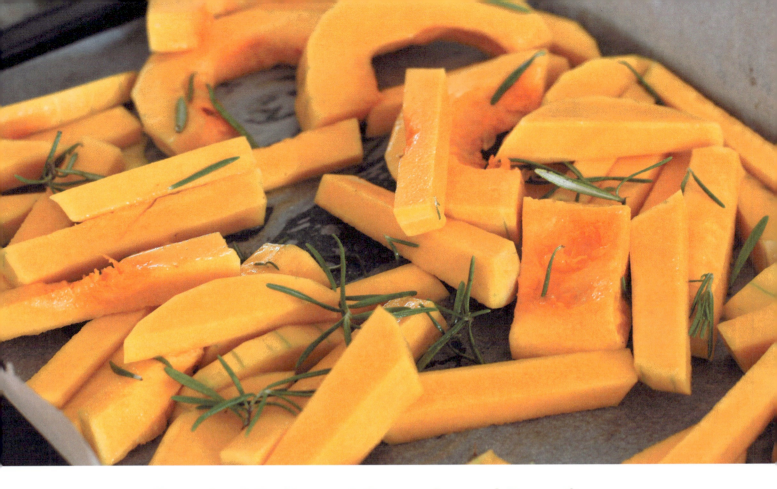

Roasted Butternut Squash and Pear Soup

1 medium butternut squash, approximately 1 pound

2 medium pears

1 medium onion, sliced

1 clove garlic, minced

2 tablespoons butter

2 cups chicken broth

1 1/2 cups almond milk

salt and pepper to taste

Directions

Preheat oven to 400 degrees.

Cut the squash in half lengthwise and scoop out the seeds. Remove the stem from each pear. Cut in half and scoop out the core.

Spray a large pan with nonstick cooking spray. Place the sliced onion, garlic, and butter on the bottom of the pan. Top with squash halves and pear halves, cut side down.

Roast 30–45 minutes until squash is cooked through and pears are soft.

Scoop flesh out of the squash and pears.

Place the flesh and remainder of the ingredients from the pan into a food processor and puree (in batches if necessary).

In a large saucepan, over medium heat, cook the broth until warm.

Add puree and cook for 10 minutes.

Lower to a simmer and add almond milk. Simmer for 8–10 minutes.

Season with salt and pepper to taste.

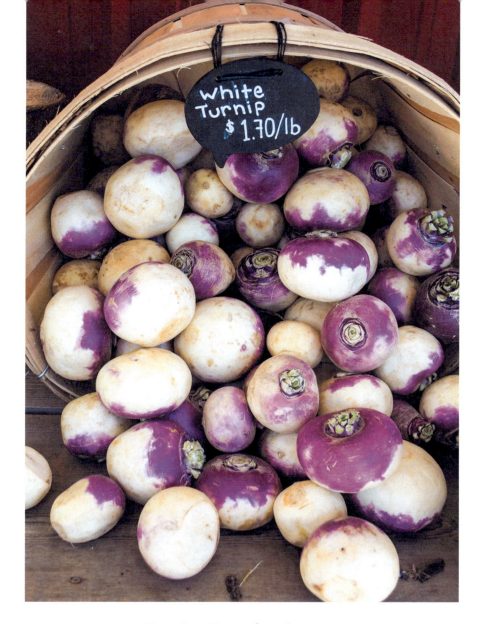

Tasty Turnip Soup

1 pound turnips, peeled and diced

1 medium sweet potato, peeled and diced

1/2 cup almond milk

3 tablespoons parsley, chopped

1/4 teaspoon red cayenne pepper (optional)

Directions

    Peel and dice turnips and sweet potato.

    Place in a large saucepan and cover with water. Bring to a boil.

    Reduce heat, cover, and simmer until tender.

    Drain, reserving a small amount of the water.

    Place vegetables in food processor or blender and puree.

    Add almond milk and cayenne. Mix again.

    Warm in saucepan with some reserved water.

    Serve with parsley sprinkled on top.

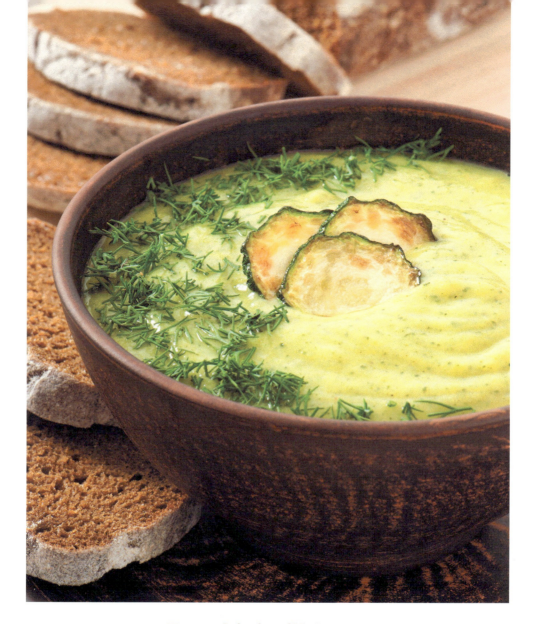

Zucchini Dill Soup

1 tablespoon olive oil

1 medium onion, diced

8 cups diced zucchini

1 teaspoon minced garlic

6 cups chicken broth

2 teaspoons dill

salt and pepper to taste

Directions

Heat oil in large saucepan over medium heat.

Add onions and sauté until tender and clear.

Add garlic and zucchini and sauté 3–4 minutes more.

Add broth, dill, salt, and pepper. Bring to a boil and cook until zucchini is tender.

Allow to cool slightly and then puree in a blender or a food processor.

Pour back into pot to warm and serve.

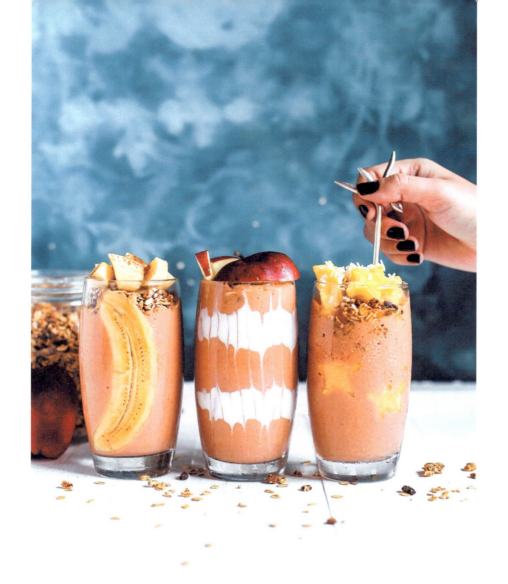

Smoothie Ingredient List

Smoothies are refreshing and hydrating. Fruits and vegetables are full of nutrients and electrolytes. Staying hydrated is necessary for healthy digestion and metabolic functioning.
You can design your own smoothie to suit your preferred flavor, while limiting refined sugars and other additives common in store-bought drinks. Follow the simple smoothie framework below and *enjoy*!

=The basic smoothie formula:

1/2–1 cup of liquid or ice (adding this first makes the smoothie blend easier)
1 cup frozen chopped fruit
1 cup fresh or frozen vegetables
up to 1/2 cup protein powder
healthy fats

Fruits

Fruit adds natural sweetness and refreshing flavor to smoothies. To avoid a sugar crash, opt for these fruits with a lower glycemic index:
- berries: strawberry, blueberry, and raspberry
- stone fruits: peach, cherry, and plum
- citrus fruits: orange, grapefruit, lemon, and lime
- pome fruits: apple and pear

Vegetables

A daily smoothie is the perfect opportunity to sneak in veggies that you won't even taste. The best vegetables for smoothies include the following.
- hydrating vegetables: zucchini, cauliflower, cucumber, and celery
- leafy greens: spinach and kale
- sweet vegetables: carrot and sweet potato

Proteins

To ensure that a smoothie is filling and keeps you full, include some protein in the blend. Great smoothie protein sources include:
- protein powders: plant-based, whey-derived, or nut powders
- sugar-free yogurt (either dairy or plant-based)
- tofu

Healthy Fats

Omega-3 fatty acids and monounsaturated fats increase satiety and heart health but are high in calories, so add these fat sources in moderation:
- nut butter
- avocado

Liquids

Use filtered water if possible or one of these hydrating liquid options to increase creaminess and flavor:
- sugar-free nut milk (coconut, almond, etc.)
- coconut water
- coffee
- tea

Extras

If desired, add extra flavor and nutrients with:
- unsweetened cocoa powder
- dried spices
- extracts like vanilla, peppermint, or coconut

Some very simple recipes for you to have in your pocket follow. Please remember to try any ingredients and add things you love.

Smoothie Tips

You will want to make sure you have the right tools for the job before preparing your smoothie. A substantial food processor or blender will do the job.

The best smoothies are well-balanced drinks with a variety of ingredients. Some smoothies can end up being a sugar drink, depending on which ingredients are included. While fruit is a great source of many vitamins, minerals, and fiber, it can also be high in sugar and carbs, especially if you're using large quantities. Regardless of whether you are diabetic, the drop in sugar afterward can feel terrible and get in the way of what you want to do during the day.

To get started, choose a liquid base, such as a nut milk. The ideal way to get a smooth smoothie is to first blend in your leafy greens with your liquid base. This is also an extremely easy way to achieve the general daily recommendation of 4–5 servings of vegetables a day. You may want to steam your veggies in advance and freeze them in appropriate portions for your recipes. Steaming helps break down fiber even more, making them easier to digest. This is good news, as we know vegetables are difficult to digest. If they are steamed and then milled in the blender, you will obviously have a much easier time digesting them. Anything that makes it easier for you, like freezing portions in ice trays or zip-top bags is a great thing.

Fresh or frozen fruit can be added next for sweetness. Fruit also provides vitamins and minerals. Healthy fats can be added to help support blood sugar balance. Fats, such as coconut oil or nut or seed butter, provide fatty acids for energy and are a source of vitamins too. Finally, add protein powder for the added amino acids (the building blocks of the body) to make the smoothie into a meal.

Make sure you balance the carbs out with ingredients that contain protein and healthy fats so the smoothie keeps you feeling energetic longer and helps you avoid a blood sugar crash. From a nutrition perspective, avocados are a good source of fiber, and unlike most fruits, they have zero grams of naturally occurring sugar per serving. Avocados are also a rich and creamy swap for typical smoothie ingredients containing saturated fats. To freeze them, simply wash, halve, peel, and quarter fresh avocados. Toss them in a resealable freezer bag for a smoothie later.

In addition to excellent protein sources like nut butters, there are protein-packed ingredients. Yogurt and kefir have probiotics, which support gut health and add a creamy element to smoothies. If you're vegan, try a vegan protein powder such as pea protein powder, which is also a great source of iron.

Simple Smoothie Recipes

Strawberry Smoothie

1 cup unsweetened milk

1 serving frozen spinach

1 cup strawberries (fresh or frozen)

1/2 cup unsweetened Greek yogurt

Chocolate Peanut Butter Smoothie

1 cup unsweetened milk

1 avocado

1 tablespoon peanut butter

1 tablespoon cocoa powder

honey or agave nectar to taste

ice

Cherry Banana Almond Smoothie

1 cup unsweetened milk

1/2 a frozen banana (or fresh banana plus ice)

1/2 cup red cherries

2 drops almond extract

Green Goddess Smoothie

1 cup unsweetened milk

1/2 cup ice

1/2 a frozen banana

1/2 cup green grapes

1 kiwi, peeled

1 cup baby spinach leaves

After blending, remove the pulp from your smoothie with a mesh strainer.

Green Apple Smoothie

1/2 cup filtered water

1 green apple peeled, cored, and diced

1/2 cucumber, peeled, deseeded, and diced

1teaspoon honey or agave nectar

2 cups baby spinach leaves

After blending, remove the pulp from your smoothie with a mesh strainer.

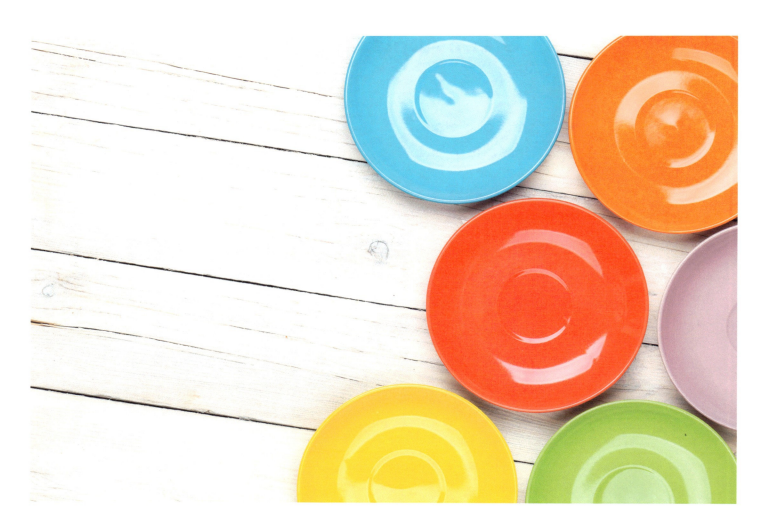

Step 3 Recipes

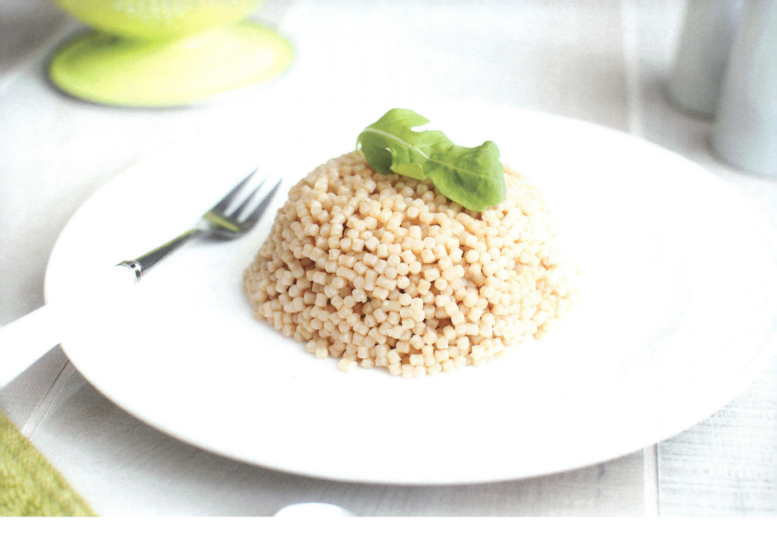

Simple Pasta

1 box acini di pepe pasta (very small)
2 cups chicken broth
1 can cream of mushroom soup
1 teaspoon parsley, finely chopped

Directions

Combine broth and soup in a saucepan and heat through.

Add pasta and cook according to directions on the box, approximately 10 minutes. Stir often and watch carefully, as the pasta is so tiny that it absorbs the liquid very quickly.

Sprinkle cooked pasta with Parmesan cheese as tolerable.

If you would find it more soothing to have more broth than pasta, do it. Add more broth and subtract pasta amounts as you please. Remember this pasta is so tiny that it absorbs liquid quickly. Stay close by as it is cooking.

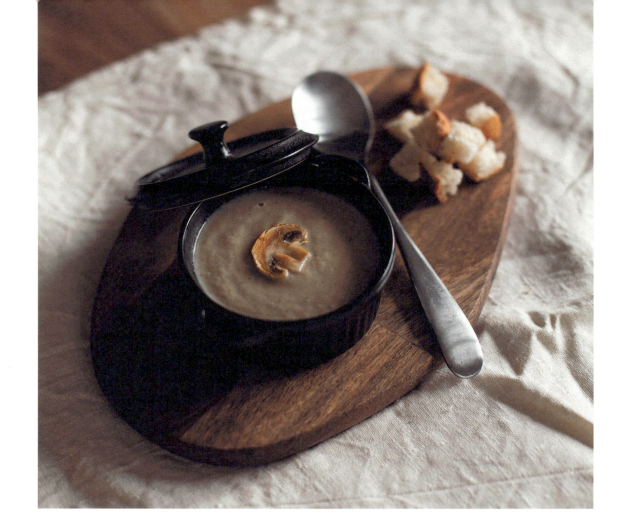

Potato and Mushroom Soup

2 cups canned or boxed mushroom soup

2 cups chicken broth

3 pounds potatoes, cut into wedges

16 ounces fresh mushrooms, chopped

salt and pepper to taste

Directions

Pour mushroom soup into large pot. Add potatoes and mushrooms and season with salt and pepper to taste.

Cover and cook over medium heat for 1 hour.

Use potato masher, blender, or food processor to smooth out the soup, depending your comfort level. We have placed this soup in step 3 because it is a hearty soup. I remember the wonderful feeling of chewing again. The soft potatoes and mushrooms were a perfect place to start solid foods again. This was one of my favorites, and I crave it as I write.

Recipe note: If this consistency is too thick for you to tolerate, add chicken broth to the point that is becomes light enough for you to eat. This recipe is a good source of protein. Potatoes are almost a perfect food and have an abundance of vitamins A, B, and C, as well as potassium.

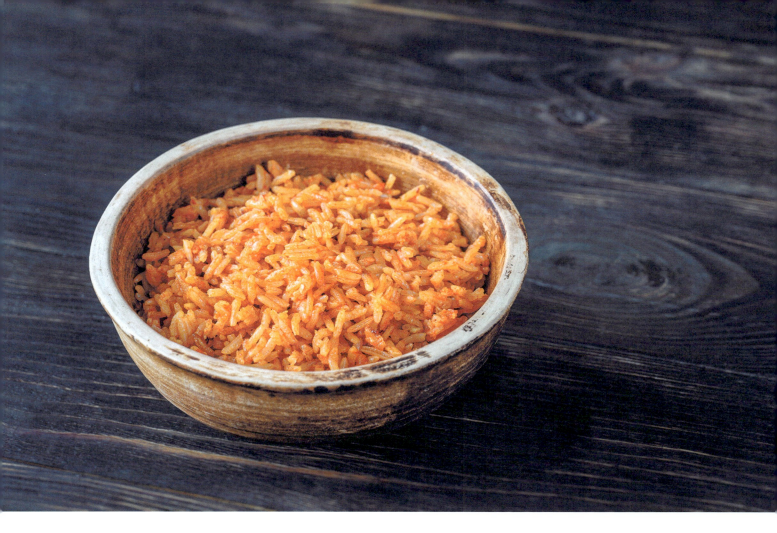

Rice Consommé

1 onion, chopped
1 stick butter
1 cup rice, uncooked
2 cans beef consommé
1 can sliced mushrooms

Directions

Preheat oven to 400 degrees.

Melt butter in a pan and sauté onion.

Add rice and brown slightly, stirring often.

Add consommé and mushrooms.

Place in 9- x13-inch baking dish and cover with foil. Bake for 30–45 minutes.

This recipe can also be used in step 2 minus the onion and mushrooms for easier digestion.

Recipe note: This recipe comes from my friend Jeanne Staples and was published in a cookbook produced by the church in which I grew up in Statesville, North Carolina, as a celebration of 250 years of worship. I have tremendous memories of nourishing food and fellowship from this sacred place and its extraordinarily loving and generous people—home. Encore: Celebrating 250 Years of First Presbyterian Church 1753–2003

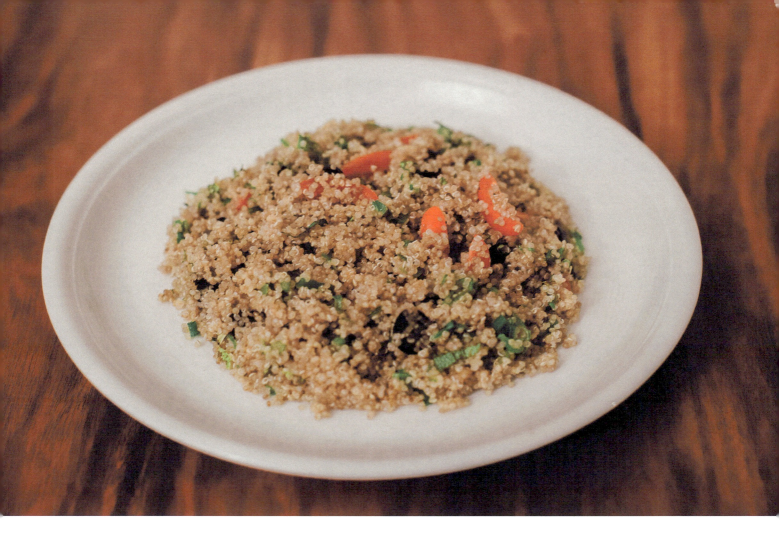

Vegetable Couscous

1 cup finely chopped mushrooms
1/2 cup finely chopped onions
1/2 cup finely chopped orange bell pepper
1/2 cup finely chopped red bell pepper
1 tablespoon olive oil
1 cup water
1 box couscous

Directions

Sauté mushrooms, onions, and bell peppers in oil until tender.
Add 1 cup water and bring to a boil.
Stir in couscous and cover.
Reduce to simmer and let stand for 5 minutes.

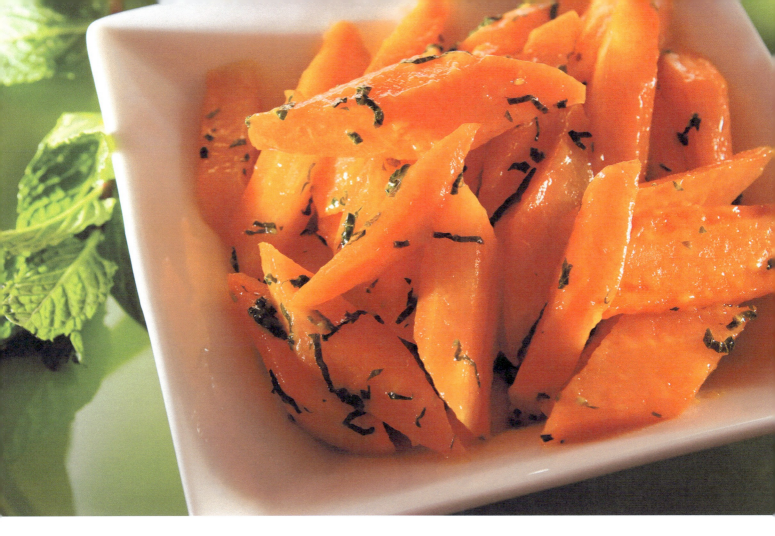

Minty Carrots

6 medium carrots, sliced
1/2 cup grapefruit juice
several sprigs of fresh mint cut into small pieces

Directions
    Steam carrots until fork tender.
    Heat grapefruit juice to boiling in a small skillet.
    Add carrots and cook over medium heat until juice is nearly evaporated, 2–3 minutes. If they are not tender enough for you, add 1/2 cup water and continue cooking until tender.
    Add mint, stir, and serve.

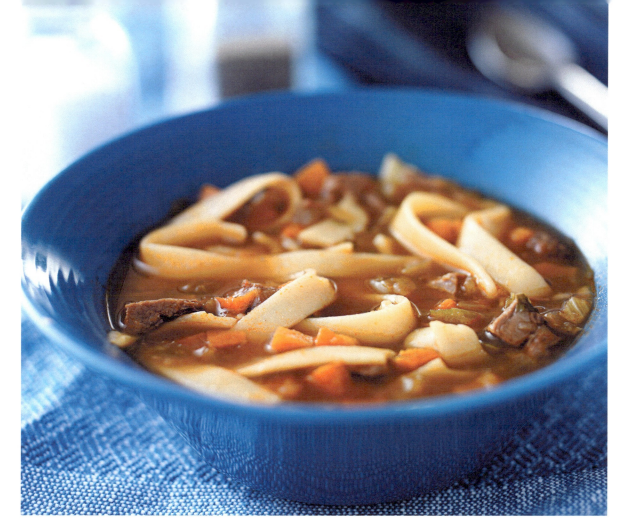

Beef Noodle Soup

1 pound lean, cubed beef stew meat (filet if you can find it)

1 cup chopped onion

1 cup chopped celery

1/4 cup beef bouillon granules

1/4 teaspoon dried parsley

1 pinch ground black pepper

5 3/4 cups water

2 1/2 cups frozen egg noodles

Directions

In a large saucepan over medium-high heat, sauté the stew meat, onion, and celery for 5 minutes, or until meat is browned on all sides. Cut into smaller pieces if this is the first time you are eating in step 3.

Stir in the bouillon, parsley, ground black pepper, carrots, water, and egg noodles.

Bring to a boil, reduce heat to low, and simmer for 30 minutes.

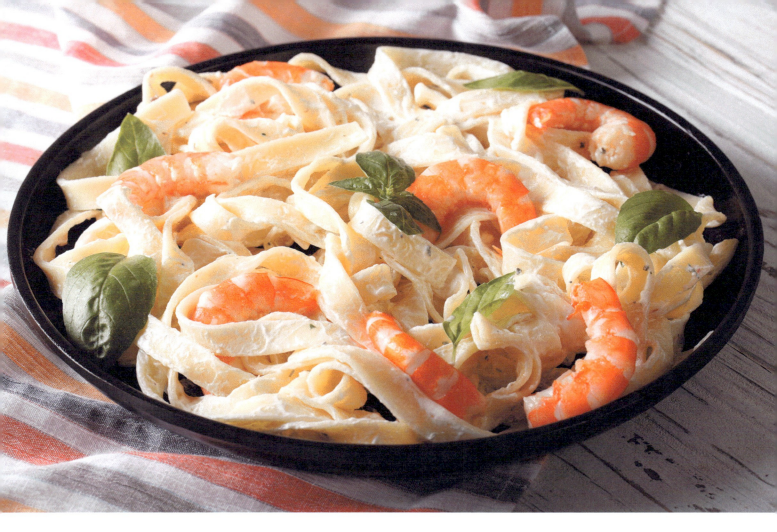

Shrimp on Fettuccine Noodles

1 pound frozen, peeled, and deveined shrimp
6 ounces fettuccine, spinach, or your favorite noodles
2 teaspoons fresh basil or 1 teaspoon dried
2 tablespoons butter

Directions

Thaw shrimp.

Prepare the fettuccine according to package directions.

In a large skillet, cook the shrimp, butter, and basil on medium heat for 2–3 minutes, or until shrimp turns pink, stirring often.

Serve over the cooked fettuccine.

Recipe note: If you are still having trouble digesting food, cut up the shrimp and pasta into smaller bites to help the process along. This is a dish that you could ask for at most restaurants. If the menu lists fettuccine alfredo, ask that the alfredo sauce be left off your dish. The key is to not have much fat or a heavy sauce. Enjoy.

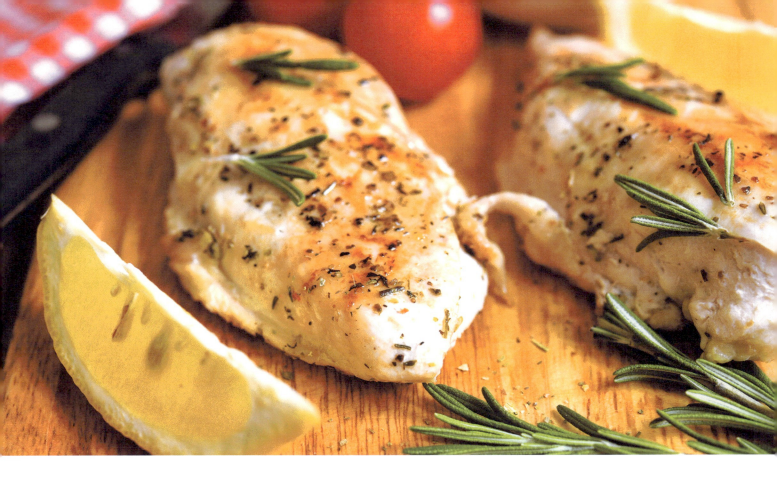

Baked Chicken Breast

Making baked, boneless chicken breasts is simple. The key is the cooking time and temperature.

Directions

Preheat the oven to 400 degrees.

Toss the chicken breasts with olive oil, herbs, and spices of your choice.

Lightly grease a baking dish and arrange chicken pieces.

Bake chicken breasts for 22–26 minutes.

Rest them before you slice or pull them.

Recipe note: Chicken breasts are mildly flavored, so you'll want to add seasonings and some salt. As most of us are often looking for a quick meal, especially when we don't feel well, you can use a marinade for flavor or your preference of seasoning. If cooked and seasoned well, chicken breasts are tender and juicy on their own. Of course, the most important thing is the flavor appeal to you. Ideas that may sound good are:

- Italian seasoning
- Cajun seasoning
- taco seasoning
- salt, pepper, olive oil, and fresh herbs with lemon zest

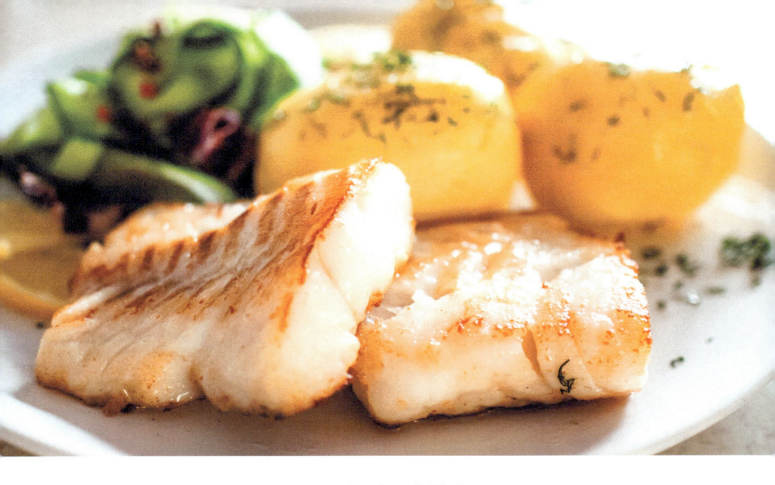

Easy Baked Fish

1 1/4 pounds fish fillets

1 teaspoon seasoned salt

pepper to taste

paprika (optional)

3 tablespoons butter, melted

Directions

Preheat oven to 400 degrees.

Place fish in a greased 11- x 7-inch baking dish.

Sprinkle with seasoned salt, pepper, and paprika if desired. Drizzle with butter.

Cover and bake until fish begins to flake easily with a fork, 15–20 minutes.

Baked Fish Tips

What's the best fish to bake? For this point in your nausea journey, you may want to choose a white fish, such as halibut, cod, bass, grouper, haddock, catfish, or snapper. White fish doesn't mean that the fish is white in color; rather, it is a mild-flavored fish that cooks quickly and seasons very well.

How can you tell when a fish is finished cooking?

To test the doneness of fish, carefully pierce the thickest portion with a fork and twist slightly to see if it flakes without resistance. If it does not, cook it longer. Make sure you are cooking fully.

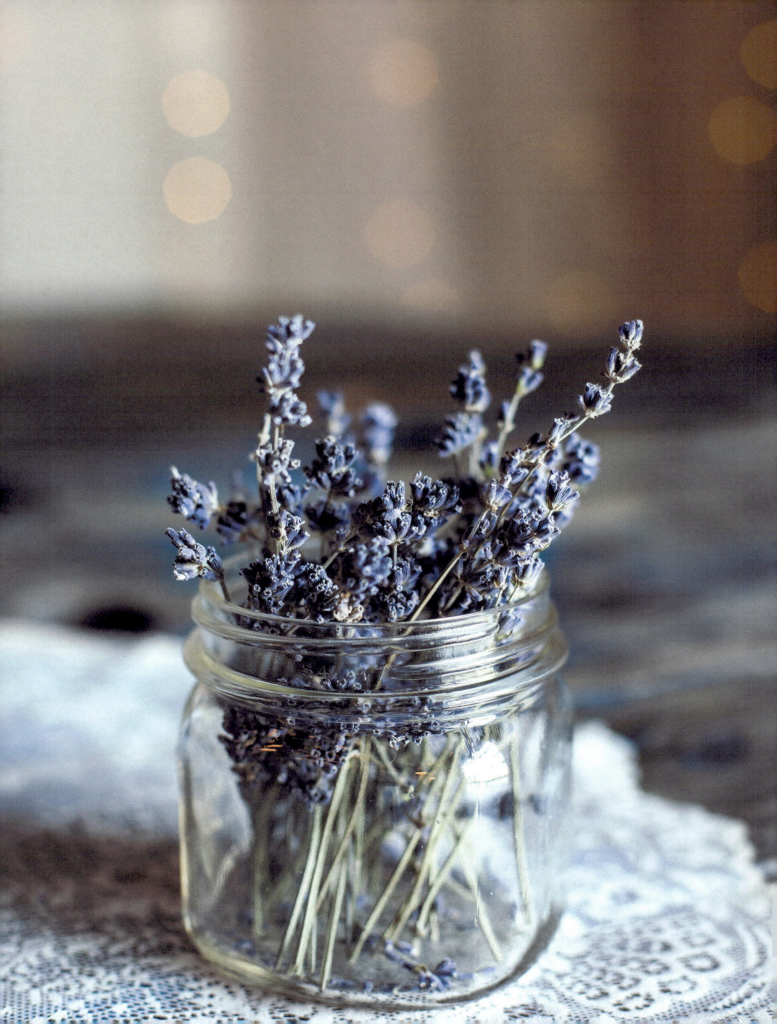

CHAPTER

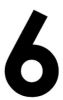

R-E-S-P-E-C-T Yourself

If you are reading this book, you are seeking answers. You are either seeking answers for yourself or someone you love. In the spirit of hope, I would like to share with you the approach I took to cope with my diagnosis of severe gastroparesis. Hopefully, sharing will help you on your own journey and encourage you to do everything you can to become well. Being diagnosed with a chronic disease can feel as if you have been dealt a paralyzing blow. This is a natural response to the unknown, yet it is key you do not remain stuck in that position.

You are in the driver's seat and must shift gears to *drive*. You are the vehicle that carries the precious cargo that is your life. We have provided a companion manual to help you understand how your vehicle, especially your digestive system, works under the hood. We have given you guidance on the best fuel for your tank. We have listed troubleshooting steps when your vehicle is not running optimally. We have also provided ways in which the cause of the problem can be determined. If your vehicle cannot be repaired now, you will need guidance on how to travel in a less-than-optimal vehicle.

There were many routes and rest areas along my journey coping with nausea and vomiting and gastroparesis. I recognize now that there were three main regions I traveled in my journey to wellness. After waiting so long to understand how my stomach and body had changed, I first had to respond to Dr. Koch's diagnosis. A ton of emotions drove me up many steep hills and into deep valleys. It was rough territory. I realized I needed to get out of there. I took a hard right. I began to repair and renovate my broken-down life by employing what I knew—interior design skills. I created a new and appropriate environment in which to park, rest, and regroup. This new environment gave me a perspective on respecting myself under these new circumstances of chronic illness. It allowed me to feel calmer and more comfortable. I was determined to do everything I could to comfort my stomach and comfort my soul.

Respond

As the uncharted journey of my illness unfolded, I responded with a roller coaster of emotions. At times, I would feel loss, sadness, anger, depression, and stress. I see now that these varying emotions were reasonable and understandable.

There was a mournful sense of loss that engulfed me. I longed for my life before my illness took over and ruled my comings and goings. I felt a renewed loss for my dear sister, Robin, and the way our lives were when we were together. She had what everyone called a difficult time living for seventeen years with the results of two ruptured brain aneurysms. Yet her larger-than-life soul embraced everything with open arms. She was the inspiration to put my life back into drive and get back on the road. If she could deal so well with her life's journey, I knew I could eventually embrace her perspective. I could learn from her even if she was no longer here. I find that is still true.

As many of Dr. Koch's patients and I have expressed, "We want our lives back." You may feel as if your life will never be the same. Sometimes there is no medical explanation or effective treatment for our symptoms. When we know the cause of our symptoms and illness, we feel we can handle it or even reverse the situation. But things do not feel OK with chronic, unexplained symptoms because you do not know how to help yourself or what to do to get your life back. Trying alternatives can be frustrating. You will learn to embrace alternatives.

Nausea and vomiting are life-altering whether they are acute or chronic. They cause changes in the way you anticipate, attend, and live life. A sense of sadness may overcome you. You are required to change and react whenever the symptoms hit. You must prepare for the unpredictable. You will find solutions.

Stress is bound to ensue when so much of your life is changing due to nausea and vomiting episodes. Feeling overwhelmed with the details of everyday life and the stress of coping is a normal response. You may not be able to support those you care about in the same way you did before your illness. New ways to care for yourself and others will become evident. You know more than you think you do. You will figure it out.

To cope with the symptoms and diagnoses, I found it important to remind myself that it is natural to have these feelings. Even if you desire to deny these feelings, I found it was more beneficial to acknowledge each of them. I needed to acknowledge and address my feelings to actively direct my journey to wellness. I found that I could respond to my illness in several ways. I suggest you do the following:

- Empower yourself with knowledge of your body and your disease or disorder.
- Ask for help from friends, family, and professionals.
- Adapt your environment to support your new needs.
- Experiment with all types of approaches to improve your symptoms and sense of well-being.

Learn

Knowledge is power. The more you know about yourself and your illness, the better you can stay in the moment and deal with it. This knowledge will empower you to make the right decisions. Read and try everything you read to nourish your body, mind, and spirit. I found it helpful to read for pleasure. Your favorite genre or writer may be comforting and might transport you to a new and entertaining place. Read everything you can that may provide direction.

Ask for Help

I suggest you develop a circle of people you can count on to help—relatives, friends, and professionals. Any time your life changes with a major medical event, you may feel a loss of control, anxiety, and uncertainty about the future. This change could certainly influence your identity and self-esteem. As this is happening to you, your family and friends see it. They are concerned for you and want to help. They may not know how to respond to the changes you are experiencing, so you need to ask them to help you and tell them what you need.

At times when you are incapacitated by your nausea and vomiting, the help of trusted friends and family may not be immediately available. I found it to be a good idea to devise a plan based on my needs and the availability of my family and friends. Your plan can include giving house keys to your most-trusted friends. Also, let them know you may notify them by texting that you need help. Be sure you have backup supplies of electrolyte-containing drinks or soups and items that are included in Dr. Koch's three-step diet. Voice-activated, Wi-Fi-powered devices connected to your locks and electrical sockets may be helpful as you plan for unexpected episodes of severe nausea and vomiting.

As I mentioned, Dr. Koch delivered my diagnosis and included, "There is no cure, but new solutions are coming all the time. I will be with you to make you as comfortable as I can." I heard his words this way: "OK, you are going to be fine. It might not always be glamorous, but we will face this together." I translated his words and his gracious tone into *hope*.

As you can imagine, these words represented a very different experience compared with what I had been going through for more than a year. I was alone in the deep, dark forest of the unknown. I was desperate to be heard. What a 180-degree difference. Dr. Koch understood and helped me understand what was going on in my body. That alone was huge relief. I went from having no idea why I was so sick, cringing as I felt people making judgements about me and my symptoms, and losing my social foundation to knowing what was going on and having a plan, at least a diet plan. That was bliss. That gave me hope. You, too, will find or have found reasons to hope along your journey to wellness.

Renovate

Renovate means to restore to a good state of repair. Of course, we use this word primarily to refer to our kitchen or bathroom. However, as we renovate our environments to improve our sense of well-being, we also are renovating ourselves.

I practice interior design. Just what is interior design and how might it contribute to your well-being? Varied notions exist about what interior design is. Many people consider interior design the application of decoration in an environment. Some think interior design is choosing colors and fabrics. Others consider interior design to be how the furniture is placed in a space. Some are fearful of the words, as they believe they have no understanding, while others assume interior design is an expensive service.

Interior design to me (not just to me, as a science) is the creation of the human experience in the built environment. Through formal education, interior designers are taught color theory, furniture construction, building code, space planning, art history, HVAC, electrical, plumbing, and lighting. This course of study in many colleges and universities is called interior architecture. Interior design that heightens human experience requires much thoughtfulness. Function is key to a well-built environment. Your daily activities—your life—should dictate the design of the environments in which you spend the most time. Each environment is different and needs special thought and consideration of all details. For example, a trip to the bathroom or refrigerator at night is more pleasant and accommodating with a night-light to keep you safe and healthy compared with blackness that can be scary and dangerous.

My knowledge of interior design was helpful in creating the new elements I knew I needed to support my altered needs when I was so ill. I describe examples of how I used these skills to make my environment support my needs below. Creating comfort and pleasure for others through interior design brings me joy like nothing else. Therefore, of course, I want to share some ideas with you on how you can help your environment to accommodate and support you!

Light

Light is profoundly pertinent to our well-being. We think of its effect in three primary ways:
- *Biologically* Light influences production of hormones that affects the sleep cycle.
- *Emotionally* Light affects mood. We all know the great feeling we get on a clear, sunny day. Some of us notice a profound mood decline in winter, which is referred to as seasonal affective disorder (SAD).
- *Visually* Light affects the ability to perform tasks. The amount of light needed depends upon the specifics of the task. Less light is required to walk around a room with which you are familiar, while reading takes more. Light level also allows us to feel safe in unfamiliar spots or situations.

Natural light is the light outdoors. This type of light is associated with improved mood, reduced eyestrain, and less fatigue. Take advantage of any natural light you have. Vitamin D levels in your system are in part a product of the sunlight you receive. It is important to many processes in your body, such as absorbing the amount of calcium you need each day. Vitamin D keeps your immune system working at optimal levels by keeping inflammation at bay. Speak with your doctor about checking your vitamin D level.

Different sources and colors of light indoors can contribute to your well-being. Like the colors of light in a rainbow, you have choices of color in most types of bulbs to meet your indoor functions. I found using lamps with full-spectrum bulbs uplifting—almost like sunlight. Full-spectrum bulbs are also available for fluorescent ceiling fixtures. When I was sick, there were not as many choices available. Experiment to see what works for you.

Sound

There are many sources of soothing sound available to you through technology. There are apps that can help put you to sleep. In general, sounds from nature are found to be most helpful to wellness. You can play nature sounds from any of your music sources. The most soothing sound in my memory was only heard at my mother's North Carolina mountain house. I remember rolling over in the dark night hearing and enjoying the sounds of rain or wind blowing through the leaves of the massive trees surrounding the house. Moving forward many years, these memories bring me a sense of safety and relaxation.

Music that inspires you is another way to fill your environment with sound for your wellness. Inspiration can come from your favorite R & B, classical, or rock artists or a playlist of multiple genres.

Being read to is another soothing sound experience. Many of us were fortunate to have our parents read to us at bedtime as children. What a pleasurable experience. Audiobooks or podcasts on topics you are curious about can be an enjoyable way to stay in touch and learn.

If you live in a noisy home or loud neighborhood, a white noise machine or air purifier will provide a din of sound to allow you to rest or relax despite the noise.

Aroma

All of us have positive and negative responses to aromas. As you know all too well, some food aromas stimulate adverse responses; other aromas are wonderful and appealing. An adverse response to aromas or smells can protect us. If you smell unexpected smoke, then you know to get yourself to safety. If what you are cooking smells odd or bad, you know not to eat it. If you smell freshly cut grass or your mother's perfume, your response may be a comforting, calming one.

You can choose what aromas you have in your environment, which is another interior design moment. Aromatherapy may support a relaxing/comforting mood you want to elicit. Consider getting a diffuser to dispense essential oils you enjoy. Certain scents and tastes are known to diminish nausea such as peppermint, ginger, spearmint, and cardamom. Lavender is also a scent that calms. I found it helpful to carry peppermint oil with me when I traveled. I applied the oil onto tissues and slowly inhaled the peppermint vapors when I felt nauseated.

Comfort

Comfort is a large notion. However, for our purposes here, I am referring to physical comfort. For instance, a comfortable seating space in your bedroom where family and friends can sit by your side, watch a movie, or play cards with you may be comforting. This was something I did for myself. I had a chair and ottoman in my bedroom so my mother could join me there in comfort. It was just wide enough for a dachshund to lie on each side of her. The whole family was happy. We had many wonderful conversations there during my illness and recovery.

Make sure your bedding is comfortable and provides comfort for you to lie down and sit up. Even adjustable bases are available for your mattress so you can alter the angle as you wish. Be sure the texture of the fabric suits you and provides the temperature your like for comfortable sleeping. If you need to purchase new bedding, choose a color that is pleasing to you. Remember that healthy sleep is important for your recovery.

Work Environment

Your workplace accommodations may have to change so you can cope with your nausea and vomiting. Depending upon your occupation, you might be able to work from home. You may need to move your desk at work to avoid nausea-provoking sights or smells. You may need more breaks for small frequent meals that your stomach can tolerate comfortably. Bring your creativity into solving these work issues so you can meet your medical needs and your responsibilities.

Respect

Well-being without self-respect is oxymoronic. To bring self-respect into your life is to accept yourself today, even though you are ill or only slowly recovering. When I was so ill, I tried anything and everything within reason to maintain my livelihood. As you know, I benefited from massage therapy, acupuncture, and yoga. There are other options you may want to try. Of course, you must proceed at your own pace and strength level. Any activity based on calming the body and soul through breathing, stretching, and strengthening your muscles is worth it.

Massage

Who doesn't love a massage? Human touch is vital, yet massage is much more than that. Professional massage may reduce the stress and anxiety that is related to your chronic symptoms. Your nausea and vomiting may result in sore muscles. Massage can help relieve the pain. Circulation can be stimulated by massage. It can also help with sleep patterns and much more.

It soon became obvious to me that massage, along with Dr. Koch's three-step diet, was most calming and therapeutic for my symptoms. During one session, I suppose I was in a state of nirvana. I had no pain, nausea, or senses. I awoke immediately to an indescribable feeling I can best say was a jolt of life and my massage therapist saying, "Whoa! Did you feel that?" She explained she had not felt any energy in my abdomen since we began our sessions. At that moment, a spark of sorts caused her hands to come up away from my skin. It was at that point my symptoms started to decrease in number and severity.

Acupuncture

Acupuncture has roots in traditional Chinese medicine. It involves inserting tiny single-use needles into the skin at specific points, depending on which system of the body is being addressed. These acupoints follow meridians or pathways through which energy (*qi*, pronounced "chee") flows. The practitioner adjusts the needles to open the pathway. In general, acupuncture stimulates the body's nervous system, which then affects physiological processes in the body. Many people seek acupuncture to relieve pain relief, deal with hormonal issues, and lessen the symptoms of autoimmune disorders. I would feel immediately better after every session I enjoyed. I always felt renewed.

Yoga

The word *yoga* comes from an ancient Sanskrit word, *yuj*, meaning "to unite" the physical, mental, and spiritual parts of you. In yoga, these parts are united in the practice of certain poses and postures. There are eight different types of yoga. Each type focuses on the breath and being in the moment of now. There are times when it is a struggle to feel the breath of future life when you feel stuck in the nausea of now. Yoga may help you to cope with your acute and chronic illness and symptoms. When I am under stress, I unconsciously hold my breath. Practicing the slow rhythmic breathing of yoga continues to help me to move forward through all life's experiences.

Living with nausea and vomiting is disruptive at the least and certainly life-altering. I hope this book will help you manage and cope with your life as you seek to comfort your stomach and calm your nausea and vomiting. Every word has been written with your best interest in mind. You can do this.

I also hope sharing my journey will help you know what you can do to nourish, flourish, and understand that you can get better. I am living thriving proof. You must participate in your journey to wellness and vow to not become the victim of this vicious disease. No way! No how! You are choosing the route your vehicle takes.

It is important for you to plan for tomorrow, next week, and next year. Your life is *not* over. Plan each day to do something that brings you joy. Ask a friend to go with you or do something by yourself that brings you a little flash of joy. Anything from an art show or a new hobby to simply sitting in your own backyard will be purposeful. The unpredictability of your nausea requires the joys of life be recognized and experienced and brought into your life as they come along. Make them happen. Have something fun to look forward to always.

You are here! You are alive! You are strong!

Resources for Support

Bibliography

Nausea and Vomiting: Diagnosis and Treatment. Eds. KL Koch, WL Hasler. Springer International Publishing, Switzerland, 2017.

Koch KL. "Gastric Neuromuscular Function and Neuromuscular Disorders." In *Sleisenger and Fordtran's Gastrointestinal and Liver Disease: Pathophysiology/Diagnosis/Management.* Eds Feldman M, Friedman LS, Brandt LJ. Elsevier, Inc., Philadelphia, 2020, pp. 735-763.

"Electrogastrography for Suspected Gastroparesis." In *Gastroparesis: Pathophysiology, Clinical Presentation, Diagnosis and Treatment.* Eds. R. McCallum, H Parkman. Elsevier, 2020..

Organizations

The American College of Gastroenterology

https://gi.org/patients/

> The ACG is the preeminent professional organization that champions the prevention, diagnosis, and treatment of digestive disorders, serving as a beacon to guide the delivery of the highest quality, compassionate, and evidence-based patient care.

The American Diabetes Association

https://www.diabetes.org

> Mission: To prevent and cure diabetes and to improve the lives of all affected by diabetes.
>
> We lead the fight against the deadly consequences of diabetes and fight for those affected by diabetes.
>
> We fund research to prevent, cure and manage diabetes.
>
> We deliver services to hundreds of communities.
>
> We provide objective and credible information.
>
> We give voice to those denied their rights because of diabetes.

The American Neurogastroenterology and Motility Society

https://motilitysociety.org

> The American Neurogastroenterology and Motility Society is an organization that was established in 1980 dedicated to the study of neurogastroenterology and gastrointestinal motility and functional GI disorders.

The Association of Gastrointestinal Motility Disorders

https://agmdhope.org
maryangela@agmdhope.org

> The Association of Gastrointestinal Motility Disorders, Inc. (AGMD) was incorporated in 1991 and is one of the oldest nonprofit organizations in existence, with a focus on digestive motility diseases and disorders. Our international organization brings together a diverse group of individuals: patients, family members, physicians, nurses, basic science and clinical researchers, pharmaceutical and diagnostic professionals, home health care workers, dietitians, biotech industrialists, other organizations and those in the community interested in digestive motility diseases and disorders.

The Gastroparesis Education Awareness and Research Society (GEAR Society)

https://theGEARsociety.org
info@theGEARsociety.org

> The GEAR Society was founded by a well gastroparesis patient to augment education for patients as well as healthcare workers, amplify awareness for the general public, and fundraise for research. In these efforts, we aim to provide a greater understanding of the insidiously devastating disease of gastroparesis.

Gastroparesis Patient Association for Cures and Treatments (G-PACT)

https://g-pact.org

> G-PACT is dedicated to increasing awareness of gastroparesis, chronic intestinal pseudo-obstruction, and colonic inertia among medical professionals, patients, and the general population. We are working toward finding a cure and/or better treatment options for people dealing with digestive tract paralysis (DTP). We provide educational resources, multiple support programs, patient advocacy programs, and other aid as needed to help patients cope and to provide hope to everyone afflicted with the condition.

International Foundation for Gastrointestinal and Disorders (IFFGD)

https://iffgd.org

> Our mission is to inform, assist, and support people affected by gastrointestinal (GI) disorders. IFFGD was founded in 1991 by one person struggling with the challenges imposed by a chronic GI disorder. Many others, from all walks of life, have joined with us. We work with patients, families, physicians, nurses, practitioners, investigators, regulators, employers, and others to broaden understanding about GI disorders, support or encourage research, and improve digestive health in the adults and children.

The Oley Foundation

https://oley.org
https://oley.org/page/contactus
518-262-5079

> Founded in 1983 by Lyn Howard, MD, and her patient, Clarence Oley Oldenburg, the Oley Foundation is a national, independent, non-profit 501(c)(3) organization that strives to enrich the lives of those living with home intravenous nutrition and tube

feeding through education, advocacy, and networking. The Foundation also serves as a resource for consumer's families, clinicians and industry representatives, and other interested parties. Programs are directed by the staff and guidance is provided by a board of dedicated professionals and patients.

The National Institutes of Health

https://www.nih.gov

> The National Institutes of Health (NIH), a part of the US Department of Health and Human Services, is the nation's medical research agency. Thanks in large part to NIH-funded medical research, Americans today are living longer and healthier. Life expectancy in the United States has jumped from 47 years in 1900 to 78 years as reported in 2009, and disability in people over age 65 has dropped dramatically in the past 3 decades. In recent years, nationwide rates of new diagnoses and deaths from all cancers combined have fallen significantly."

The Gastroparesis Clinical Research Consortium

https://jhuccs1.us/gpcrc/default.asp

> The Gastroparesis Clinical Research Consortium is sponsored by the National Institute of Diabetes and Digestive and Kidney Diseases (NIDDK) to focus on the etiology, natural history, and therapy of gastroparesis. The goal of this consortium is to perform clinical, epidemiological, and therapeutic research in gastroparesis and provide an infrastructure that can rapidly and efficiently design and conduct clinical trials for effective medical, surgical, or other interventions to improve treatment of patients with gastroparesis.

Quaintance-Weaver Restaurants & Hotels

www.qwrh.com

qwrhinfo@qwrh.com

> Our grounding on the idea of being of genuine service to others makes us different from most other companies. QW is built on the idea that it is a worthwhile objective to be of genuine service to the communities we touch. We believe that if we really get the "rubber to the road" with this worthwhile objective of genuine service, then financial sustainability and an organization-wide sense of accomplishment will be the natural by-products. We are also unusual because QW is owned by its staff.

Glossary of Terms

acute – Describes an illness of sudden onset that lasts no more than two or three days.

adrenal glands – Make cortisol, a stress hormone. The glands are located above the kidneys.

adrenal insufficiency – Occurs when the adrenal glands do not make enough cortisol. Addison's disease is one specific type of this insufficiency.

alcohol poisoning (intoxication) – A serious consequence of drinking large amounts of alcohol in a short period of time. Drinking too much too quickly can affect your breathing, heart rate, body temperature, and gag reflex. These effects can potentially lead to coma and death.

amylase – An enzyme secreted by the salivary glands and the pancreas that converts starch into simple sugars.

amyotrophic lateral sclerosis (ALS) – A progressive nervous system disease that affects nerve cells in the brain and spinal cord, causing loss of muscle control. ALS is also called Lou Gehrig's disease after the baseball player who was diagnosed with it.

anal sphincters – Rings of muscle at the opening of the anus. The internal and external sphincters keep the anus closed as stool collects in the rectum.

anorexia nervosa – A psychiatric disorder characterized by markedly reduced appetite or total aversion to food. The cycle of restrictive eating may lead to starvation and death.

antrectomy – The surgical resection of the antrum.

antrum – The part of the stomach that mixes and mills the food we eat and empties the milled food (called chyme) into the duodenum.

appendix – A tube-shaped organ that is attached to the cecum of the colon. If it becomes inflamed (i.e., appendicitis) it is removed (i.e., appendectomy).

ascending colon – The section of the colon between the cecum and transverse colon. This part of colon absorbs much of the liquid that is emptied into it from the ileum.

autonomic nervous system (ANS) – The part of the nervous system that controls involuntary functions such as digestion, blood pressure, and respiration.

bile – A fluid made by the liver and stored in the gallbladder that aids in digestion and nutrient absorption.

body (corpus) of the stomach – This forms the lower half of the stomach with the antrum. The body and antrum mix and mill the food we eat into chyme, which is emptied from the stomach into the duodenum.

bradygastria – An abnormally slow gastric electrical rhythm that ranges from 1.0–2.5 cycles per minute.

bulimia – A psychiatric disorder associated with self-induced vomiting and purging of food. Laxatives and diuretics are sometimes abused to rid the body of food that has been recently ingested.

CAT (computerized axial tomography) scan – Produces detailed images of structures inside the body, such as organs of the digestive and reproductive tract, blood vessels, and bones.

cecum – Forms the first part of the large intestine and is connected to the ileum by the ileocecal valve. The cecum receives liquids from the ileum and moves them into the ascending colon.

central nervous system (CNS) – The part of the nervous system that consists of the brain and spinal cord. The brain processes and responds to sensory and hormonal information from the spinal cord, cranial nerves, and blood vessels.

chronic – Describes an illness that lasts from weeks to years.

chyme – Finely milled food ready for emptying from the antrum into the duodenum.

colon – The digestive tract organ responsible for absorbing liquid emptied into it from the ileum, harboring the microbiome (bacteria of the colon), and concentrating foodstuffs that cannot be absorbed into stool. The formed stool is eliminated through the anus during bowel movements.

coronavirus – A common virus that causes infections in the nose, sinuses, or throat. Most coronaviruses aren't dangerous. However, in early 2020, after a December 2019 outbreak in China, the World Health Organization identified SARS-CoV-2 as a new type of coronavirus. The outbreak quickly became a devastating worldwide pandemic.

cortisol – A stress hormone released from the adrenal glands.

cholecystectomy – The operation to remove the gallbladder because of symptoms caused by gallstones or dysfunction in gallbladder emptying.

cholecystokinin (CCK) – A hormone that is secreted by cells in the duodenum and stimulates contraction of the gallbladder to empty bile through the bile duct and into the duodenum. CCK also stimulates secretion of digestive enzymes by the pancreas.

dehydration – Occurs when the body loses water and electrolytes like sodium and potassium due to excess sweating, vomiting, or diarrhea. Dehydration can lead to light-headedness, fainting, and more severe medical conditions.

descending colon – The part of the colon on the left side of the abdomen that connects the transverse colon to the sigmoid colon. The descending colon holds stool for further processing by the microbiome.

diabetes mellitus (DM) – A disease that results in abnormally high blood glucose levels due to insufficient insulin in type 1 diabetes and insulin resistance in type 2 diabetes.

disease – A condition of the living animal or of one of its parts that impairs normal function and is typically manifested by signs and symptoms.

disorder – A disturbance of normal functioning of the mind or body that may be caused by genetic factors, diseases, or trauma. There may not be enough measurable abnormalities or specific clinical evidence for a disorder to be called a disease.

duodenum – The first part of the small intestine that receives the bits of milled food (chyme) that are emptied through the pylorus located at the end of the stomach.

dyspepsia – Means "bad digestion" and encompasses the symptoms of upper abdominal discomfort, easy filling, prolonged fullness, nausea, and vomiting after ingestion of food.

E. coli (*Escherichia coli*) – A bacterium that occurs in various strains. It may live as harmless inhabitants of the colon or may produce a toxin causing diarrhea.

EGD (esophagogastroduodenoscopy) or upper endoscopy – A procedure during which a flexible fiber-optic instrument (called an endoscope) is used to examine the lining of the esophagus, stomach, and duodenum. Several therapies can be performed with the endoscope during an upper endoscopy procedure.

electrogastrogram (EGG) – A record of gastric myoelectrical activity measured with electrodes placed on the surface of the abdomen.

electrogastrography – The method for measuring the electrical rhythms of the stomach. These recordings are called electrogastrograms (EGGs). They are like EKGs, which measure the heart's electrical rhythms, and EEGs, which measure the brain's electrical rhythms.

electrolytes – Minerals like sodium and potassium that are present in the blood. They are measured in standard blood tests.

endocrine system – Includes glands that produce and secrete hormones directly into the bloodstream. For example, cortisol (a stress hormone) is secreted from the adrenal gland, and thyroxine (a hormone that helps regulate metabolism) is secreted from the thyroid gland.

enteric nervous system (ENS) – A separate nervous system within the gastrointestinal tract that controls secretions and neuromuscular activity. The autonomic nervous system (ANS) and central nervous system (CNS) interact with the ENS to help control gastrointestinal functions.

enterotoxins – Toxic products of bacteria that cause diarrhea.

enzymes – Proteins that activate or inhibit cellular metabolism. Enzymes are needed to make building blocks of the cells or help break down other substances.

epiglottis – A flap of cartilage at the root of the tongue, which is depressed during swallowing to cover the larynx, opening to the trachea, or windpipe.

esophagitis – Inflammation of the lining cells of the esophagus.

esophagus – The muscular tube that connects the bottom of the throat to the top of the stomach or fundus. The esophagus transfers swallowed food to the stomach.

eugastria – The normal stomach electrical rhythm that ranges from 2.5–3.7 cycles per minute (cpm) and averages 3 cpm.

exocrine – Refers to glands that secrete their products through ducts into other organs (like saliva secreted from salivary glands into the mouth).

falciform ligament – A thin, fibrous ligament that separates the two lobes of the liver.

food poisoning – Occurs after the ingestion of food contaminated with toxins or bacteria and results in abdominal pain and diarrhea.

fundoplication – A surgical procedure during which the fundus is wrapped around the lower part of the esophagus as a treatment for heartburn.

fundus – The upper region of the stomach that is connected to the esophagus at the lower esophageal sphincter. As food is swallowed, the fundus relaxes to accommodate the food as it first enters the stomach.

gallbladder – The small, pear-shaped organ beneath the liver. Bile made by the liver is stored in the gallbladder before it is released into the duodenum.

gallstones – Crystalline masses in the gallbladder or bile ducts formed from bile, cholesterol, calcium, or other salts. Gallstones can cause inflammation and thus pain when they block the cystic duct or common bile duct.

gastric dysrhythmias – The abnormal electrical rhythms of the stomach that reflect disturbances in the normal stomach pacemaker rhythm (e.g., bradygastrias and tachygastrias).

gastric emptying test – A procedure to determine the rate of emptying of a test meal, usually a solid meal. A small amount of radioactive material is cooked in scrambled egg replacement. The rate of emptying of the meal from the stomach can then be measured by a special camera that detects the amount of meal in the stomach over time.

gastric neuromuscular dysfunction – Refers to abnormalities in stomach muscle relaxation, contraction, and electrical rhythm. Dysfunction in one or all these activities can result in symptoms after ingestion of food, gastric dysrhythmias, and gastroparesis.

gastric ulcers – Craters of inflammation in the lining of the stomach due to stomach acid, anti-inflammatory drugs (e.g., ibuprofen), or the bacteria H. pylori.

gastritis – Inflammation of the lining of the stomach.

gastroenteritis – Inflammation of the lining of the stomach and small intestine.

gastrointestinal hormones – Special molecules released into the blood that affect digestive functions.

gastroparesis – Paralysis or weakness of the stomach defined by delayed emptying of a test meal. The severity of stomach paralysis varies from mild to severe.

glucagon – A hormone that increases blood glucose by stimulating glycogen breakdown in the liver and muscles.

glucose – A crucial nutrient required by the body for metabolism and energy.

glycogen – A complex form of glucose that is stored in the liver and muscles.

H_2 receptor blockers – Medicines that reduce the amount of acid produced by the acid secreting cells (parietal cells) in the lining of the stomach.

Helicobacter pylori (H. pylori) – A bacterium that causes peptic ulcers, gastritis, and stomach cancer.

hepatic artery – The main blood vessel that supplies the liver with oxygenated blood.

hepatic portal vein – The blood vessel that carries blood from the gastrointestinal tract, gallbladder, pancreas, and spleen to the liver.

hormone – Represents signaling molecules produced in endocrine glands and transported through the bloodstream to distant organs to regulate physiology and behavior.

hyperemesis gravidarum – Prolonged, severe nausea and vomiting that occurs during pregnancy and may lead to weight loss and dehydration.

hyperthyroidism – The excessive release of thyroxine from the thyroid gland.

hypothyroidism – The insufficient release of thyroxine from the thyroid gland.

idiopathic – Denotes any disease or condition for which the cause is unknown.

ileum – The last region of the small intestine and connects the jejunum and the cecum of the colon.

ileocecal valve – A sphincter positioned at the joining of the ileum and the cecum. It helps to regulate the flow of liquid contents from the ileum into the cecum.

immunity – Provided by special cells located in the blood and tissues that protect us from viruses, bacteria, parasites, and other foreign material as appropriate to maintain health.

influenza – An acute, highly contagious respiratory disease caused by A, B, or C orthomyxoviruses.

indigestion – Feeling bad after a meal with the onset of nausea, excessive fullness, bloating, and abdominal discomfort.

insulin – A hormone released from the pancreas into the bloodstream that lowers blood glucose.

interstitial cells of Cajal (ICC) – The pacemaker cells of the gastrointestinal system that control, or pace, the frequency and movement of contractions, called peristaltic contractions. In the stomach, the pacemaker frequency is normally three cycles per minute. ICC were described by Santiago Ramon y Cajal, a Spanish neuroscientist, pathologist, and histologist who won the Nobel Prize in Physiology/Medicine in 1906.

ischemia – A deficient supply of blood to a body part due to obstruction of the inflow of arterial blood or outflow of venous blood.

jejunum – The middle region of the small intestine. The duodenum comes before the jejunum, and then the jejunum transitions to the ileum, which is the last anatomical region of the small intestine. The jejunum absorbs the tiny particles of food broken down by digestion. These particles or nutrients include glucose, amino acids and fatty acids.

L-dopa – The form of dopa that is obtained from fava beans or prepared synthetically. It is converted to dopamine, an important neurotransmitter, in the brain and is used in treating Parkinson's disease.

lipase – An enzyme secreted from the pancreas into the duodenum to break down triglycerides to fatty acids, a form of fat that can be absorbed in the small intestine.

liver – A large organ that produces many proteins from the nutrients absorbed in the jejunum and ileum. The liver stores carbohydrates in the form of glycogen, metabolizes drugs, produces bile, and secretes it into the gallbladder.

lower esophageal sphincter – A ring of smooth muscle located between the end of the esophagus and fundus of the stomach. When the lower esophageal sphincter is closed, it prevents acid and stomach contents from backing up (refluxing) into the esophagus.

metabolism – Represents the many chemical reactions in the cells of the body that change food into energy. Our bodies need this energy for life to do everything from moving to thinking to growing.

meningitis – Inflammation of the meninges of the brain caused by viral or bacterial infection. It is marked by intense headache and fever, sensitivity to light, nausea and vomiting, and a very stiff neck. Meningitis in severe cases may progress to convulsions, delirium, and death.

microbiome – Refers to the billions of bacteria in the colon that help break down the indigestible fibers that we eat. The microbiome also has a role in regulation of the immune system and protects us from bad bacteria that cause disease. It produces vitamins B12, thiamine, riboflavin, and vitamin K.

migraine – A type of headache associated with dilation of blood vessels in the head.

mixed gastric dysrhythmia – An abnormal electrical rhythm of the stomach that has elements of bradygastria and tachygastria.

morning sickness – Nausea that occurs in the first trimester of pregnancy.

motion sickness – Nausea and vomiting that occurs when the body experiences noxious and stressful movements (e.g., a bumpy flight) or the illusion of motion (e.g., virtual reality googles).

muscular dystrophy – A group of diseases that cause progressive weakness and loss of muscle mass particularly in the legs and hips. Abnormal genes interfere with the production of proteins needed to relax and contract striated muscles. Some patients have gastroparesis.

myopathic – Refers to diseases that affect the smooth, striated, or cardiac muscles.

narcotics – Drugs for pain. However, they also dull the senses and induce drowsiness. In excessive amounts, addiction or overdoses narcotics cause failure of respiration, coma, convulsions, and death.

neurogastroenterology – The specialty within gastroenterology that focuses on neuromuscular function of the gastrointestinal tract, particularly disorders and diseases of the esophagus, stomach, small intestine, colon, and rectum. Neurogastroenterology also encompasses study of the hunger, satiety, and integration of CNS, ANS, and ENS.

neurogenic – Means caused, controlled, or arising in the nervous system.

neuromuscular – Refers to both nerve and muscle.

neuropathic – Refers to damage, disease, or dysfunction of nerves, especially of the peripheral nervous system. Neuropathic pain can include burning or shooting pain but also numbness or tingling sensations.

nonsteroidal anti-inflammatory drugs (NSAIDs) – A class of medication that reduces pain, fever, and inflammation.

opioids – Narcotic drugs used to treat severe pain. The drugs include morphine, oxycodone, hydrocodone, fentanyl, and tramadol. The illegal drug heroin is morphine derived from opium poppy plants. All opioids are addictive.

pancreas – A large gland located behind the stomach. The pancreas produces and secretes digestive enzymes into the duodenum. Embedded in the pancreas are the islets of Langerhans, which secrete the hormones insulin and glucagon into the bloodstream.

pancreatitis – A disease in which the pancreas becomes inflamed. Passage of gallstones through the common bile duct may cause pancreatitis.

parasympathetic nervous system (PNS) – The part of the nervous system that slows the heart rate and breathing rate. This system also modulates the secretions and neuromuscular activities of the digestive system.

Parkinson's disease – A progressive nervous system disorder that affects limb movement and swallowing. Symptoms start gradually with a barely noticeable tremor in a hand but commonly progresses to stiffness, weakness, and slowing of movement or gait.

peptic ulcer disease (PUD) – Occurs when ulcers (inflamed craters) develop in the lining of the stomach or duodenum. Ulcers may cause pain or bleeding. Peptic ulcer disease develops because stomach acid or a bacterial infection (H. pylori) destroys the protective lining of stomach or duodenum. People who frequently take NSAIDs often develop ulcers.

peripheral nervous system (PNS) – Refers to the nervous system containing nerve cell bodies located outside of the central nervous system (CNS). The PNS is divided in the autonomic nervous system (ANS) and the enteric nervous system (ENS). The ANS is composed of the sympathetic and parasympathetic nervous systems and the ENS is the nervous system within the gastrointestinal tract. The primary role of the PNS is to transmit information from the organs, limbs, and skin to the CNS and to transmit motor (i.e., action or excitatory information) from the CNS to the peripheral organs.

peristaltic waves – Ring-like contractions of the stomach that migrate from the corpus through the antrum and stop or fade away at the pylorus. These are peristaltic contractions that occur at rate of three contractions per minute, the gastric pacemaker frequency. Peristaltic contractions also occur in the small intestine and colon.

physiology – The branch of biology that deals with the normal functions of living organisms and their many systems.

postural orthostatic tachycardia syndrome (POTS) – A condition that affects blood pressure regulation. POTS may cause light-headedness, fainting, and an uncomfortable, rapid increase in heartrate. These symptoms begin after standing up from a reclining position and are relieved by sitting or lying down.

proteases – Enzymes that break down proteins and peptides.

proton pump inhibitors (PPIs) – Drugs that inhibit the enzyme that helps produce acid in the parietal cells in the lining of the stomach. PPIs are used to treat acid related diseases like esophagitis, gastritis, and ulcers.

pylorus – A ring of smooth muscle, a sphincter, at the end of the antrum that functions as a valve to regulate the flow of stomach contents or chyme into the duodenum.

pyloroplasty – An operation during which the pylorus is cut if it is deformed by scar tissues and is the cause of delayed gastric emptying. Some patients with delayed gastric emptying or gastroparesis have neuromuscular dysfunction of the pylorus and pyloric therapies include balloon dilation, injection of Botox, or pyloroplasty.

Roux-en-Y – An operation during which most of the stomach is removed to treat cancer or nonhealing ulcers. The remaining stomach, the fundus, is connected to the jejunum. The operation is also called the gastric bypass operation when it is performed to treat morbid obesity. In this operation, the bypassed portion of the stomach is not removed.

salivary glands – Glands that make saliva. Saliva contains enzymes that begin the process of digesting food. Saliva also contains antibodies and other substances that help prevent infections of the mouth and throat.

salmonella – A bacterium spread by the fecal-oral route that may cause severe diarrhea.

Shy-Drager syndrome – A progressive disorder of the central and sympathetic nervous systems, also called multiple system atrophy. Initial symptoms may include blackouts, constipation, impotence in men, and urinary incontinence. Later symptoms are impaired speech, difficulties with breathing and swallowing, and inability to sweat.

shigella – A bacterium and intestinal pathogen that causes dysentery. The genus is named after Kiyoshi Shiga, who first discovered it in 1897.

sigmoid colon – The S-shaped section of the colon positioned between the descending colon and the rectum.

small intestine – The portion of the GI tract between the stomach and colon that is composed of three regions: the duodenum, the jejunum, and the ileum.

smooth muscle – The muscle of the gastrointestinal tract, bladder, and blood vessels. Smooth muscle is considered involuntary muscle because it contracts and relaxes without your control. That is, it works automatically.

stomach – The organ that receives and mixes solid food into chyme and then empties it in a carefully regulated manner into the duodenum. The stomach has anatomical regions called the fundus, corpus, antrum, and pylorus.

stomach contractile activity – Contractions of the smooth muscle of the stomach.

striated muscle – The muscle in biceps, thighs, and other areas that you can voluntarily contract or relax, like when you work out with bar bells.

sympathetic nervous system (SNS) – The fight-or-flight part of the nervous system that is activated during stress or dangers. The stomach has many innervations from the sympathetic nervous system.

tachygastria – An abnormally rapid gastric electrical rhythm from 3.7–10.0 cycles per minute (cpm).

trachea – A tube reinforced by rings of cartilage, extending from the larynx to the bronchial tubes. It conveys air to and from the lungs.

transverse colon – The region of the colon between the ascending colon and the descending colon. The transverse colon passes across the abdomen and usually below the level of the stomach. It can absorb liquids but also move more solid contents into the descending colon for further work by the microbiome.

triglycerides – The main constituents of natural fats and oils.

traumatic brain injury (TBI) – A physical injury to the head that affects brain functions.

upper esophageal sphincter – A ring of striated muscle located at the top of esophagus and below the root of the tongue. This sphincter opens but then closes very quickly after each swallow so any content in the esophagus cannot reflux back into the throat and result in aspiration into the trachea and lungs.

vagotomy – An operation during which the vagus nerve is cut to decrease gastric acid production. The vagus nerve is a cranial nerve that connects the brain with the stomach and other areas of the digestive tract.

vagus nerve – One of the twelve cranial nerves. It controls secretions and neuromuscular activity in the gastrointestinal tract.

virus – A tiny collection of genetic code (RNA and DNA) wrapped in a protein coat. Viruses can only reproduce and multiply within the living cells of a host.

Printed in the United States
by Baker & Taylor Publisher Services